When Hope Declines

Thoughts, experiences, and suggestions on care giving from a caregiver

©2022 T.L. McBride
All rights reserved.
ISBN 979-8-848-25886-8
2nd Edition

No part of this book may be produced in any form whatsoever without written permission except in the case of brief passages in critical reviews and articles.

Original graphics by T.L. McBride

Dedication

This book is dedicated to everyone who either is currently, has been, or will be a caretaker. No matter how much or how little time is spent in the care of others, it is sometimes difficult, but it is always valuable, necessary and worth your time. I appreciate you, the reader, selecting this book from the sea of books regarding caretaking. It is my hope that you will find it valuable and worth your time.

To all those who read this book before it was published, I very much appreciate your collective wisdom and the sharing of your opinions and insights, helping me to make this better. Life is all about people and I consider myself very lucky to have the people in my life that I do. Remember to enjoy the people in your life and live each day to the fullest. Thanks for reading......

Contents

Chapter One — 1
    About Me
    What is Caregiving?

Chapter Two — 6
    My Caregiving Start
    Understanding the Medical Industry

Chapter Three — 19
    Mobility Aids
    Ramps-Walkers-Chairs
    Bathrooms-Vision

Chapter Four — 36
    Ron's Diagnosis
    Treatments/Expectations

Chapter Five — 50
    Hospice
    Funerals
    Stuff
    Financial Concerns

Chapter Six — 67
    Back to the Mom
    Drug Costs and Concerns
    Rehab Center

Chapter Seven — 86
    Senior Care Suggestions
    Gadgets & Gizmos
    Dementia
    Hospice

Chapter Eight — 101
    Burnout
    Empathy vs' Compassion
    Final Days
    Logistics

Chapter Nine — 113
    Hindsight
    Dog Gone It

Chapter Ten — 120
    Final Thoughts
    Suggested Reading
    Links

Chapter One

A Little About Me

I am not a writer, not a medical professional, or even a college graduate, so why am I writing this book? Life has showered me with some experiences I never expected to go through and this knowledge or these insights learned from being a caregiver for two family members, I would like to share with fellow caregivers.

Do I have some life or soul saving answers to save you from the mental and physical toll that a caregiver goes through? Nope. Do I think I have a perspective that might help, some ideas that you might not have thought of, and some hindsight knowledge that could save you a tiny bit of stress as you walk this road of care and responsibility for someone else? I think, perhaps, so. Having said that, I do want to be clear that all that I have written is from my perspective. There is never only one way or path in life, so I encourage you to do your own research, make your own decisions, and provide care the way it works best for you and your loved one(s).

Over the last few years, I have had the "responsibility" of taking care of a brother and mother for their end-of-life experiences as well as viewing friends going through similar situations. My two "patients" were different, but one similarity was that at some point they both said, "There is no hope." This of course is where I came up with the title for this book. I hope I personally never get to that point, but perhaps we all will if we are lucky enough to make it to our golden years. Well, that is what some people call those years anyway. I think if you talk to anyone past prime, they will tell you there isn't a damn thing golden about it. Later I will discuss "hope" in more detail.

My biggest lesson learned and most difficult to implement is that you should enjoy life now no matter your age. Don't assume that you have time in the future or when this or that happens then you will take some time or after someone dies you will begin to enjoy your life. None of us know that we will have longevity or that if you do, you will be in good enough health to enjoy anything. If you are not enjoying your life now or doing things that make you happy or bring you joy, MAKE SOME CHANGES!

This Book

This isn't a biography of dying people or an autobiography about me. However, I have chosen to detail historical information about people so that you might have a context about where I am coming from and the background of the people I was responsible for taking care of. Dates are difficult for me, and I don't think they are relevant to anyone else or their situation, so I am not going to bother with specific months or years, only the timeline in regards to medical care and decline. The goal is to bring up topics as they appeared for me and hopefully offer some insights for you.

If you are anything like me, which you just might be or you wouldn't have found this book, you like to have answers. I read books on caretaking, but I didn't find them to be helpful for my situation. This is why I have taken the time to write this book. If I have done a good job, maybe it could be viewed as a manual to guide others through this process. As you know, life is full of lessons, some fun and some real shit sandwiches. If I can save you from a few of those sandwiches, then I have been successful.

Responsibility; Why am I in Charge?

I was always the quiet kid in the back of the class. Why? Because I didn't want to draw attention to myself. I was definitely NOT an outgoing, take-charge sort of person. So why did I find myself in charge of others well-being? It seems that some people are just not very good at managing their lives and certainly not when it comes to health issues. I on the other hand over-think, over-analyze, organize, and to-do list myself to the nth degree. So, guess who ends up in charge? I never wanted to be in charge of anyone. I chose not to have children. I chose to have a dog and as everyone knows, they are in charge of you. (Unless you are Cesar Millan). At first, I was frustrated about being "the boss," but now I realize they needed me because on their own, they just didn't know what to do. And really, in retrospect, I was honored to have that job. It breaks my heart to think of all the people who have no one to help through a difficult health crisis or during the potentially hellish final days. Worse yet, all those with abusive family members or paid caregivers that should choose a different profession. So, no matter how heart wrenching, physically demanding, or soul sucking caregiving can be, I was grateful for the opportunity.

What is Caregiving?

I have a Webster's dictionary from the 60's. Apparently, it wasn't even a word at that time. The closest was "Caretaker: one put in charge of anything." It is an official word now. Caregiver is: a person who provides direct care (as for children, elderly people, or the chronically ill). Another definition from the freedictionary.com: a lay individual who assumes responsibility for the physical and emotional needs of another who is incapable of self-care. That might be a better definition. All that is semantic and obvious. What you might not know is although statistics vary, 30% or more of caregivers die before the person or persons they are taking care of. Sure, many of those were also perhaps in need of a caregiver. But what you will find to be very difficult during the caregiving process is taking care of yourself. As they say when flying, put your face mask on first. (And no, that has nothing to do with Covid19.) Bottom line, it is really a difficult job, role, calling or whatever you want to term it and it has no clear path or job description.

Also, there are many types of caregivers, and all are valuable. A friend of mine who happens to be in the senior stage of life, lives in a mobile home park which is home to many other seniors. Unfortunately, many are what might be termed shut in. They no longer drive, find it difficult to be mobile and many live alone. My friend visits with them, drives them to the store, helps them with home repairs, takes them food, etc. Some of these people do have relatives that help them but many of them do not and have no human interaction for days on end. After reading my book my friend said, "I wouldn't be a great caregiver, I couldn't do what you did." To which I replied, "That's just it, you are a caregiver, and your neighbors are lucky to have you in their lives."

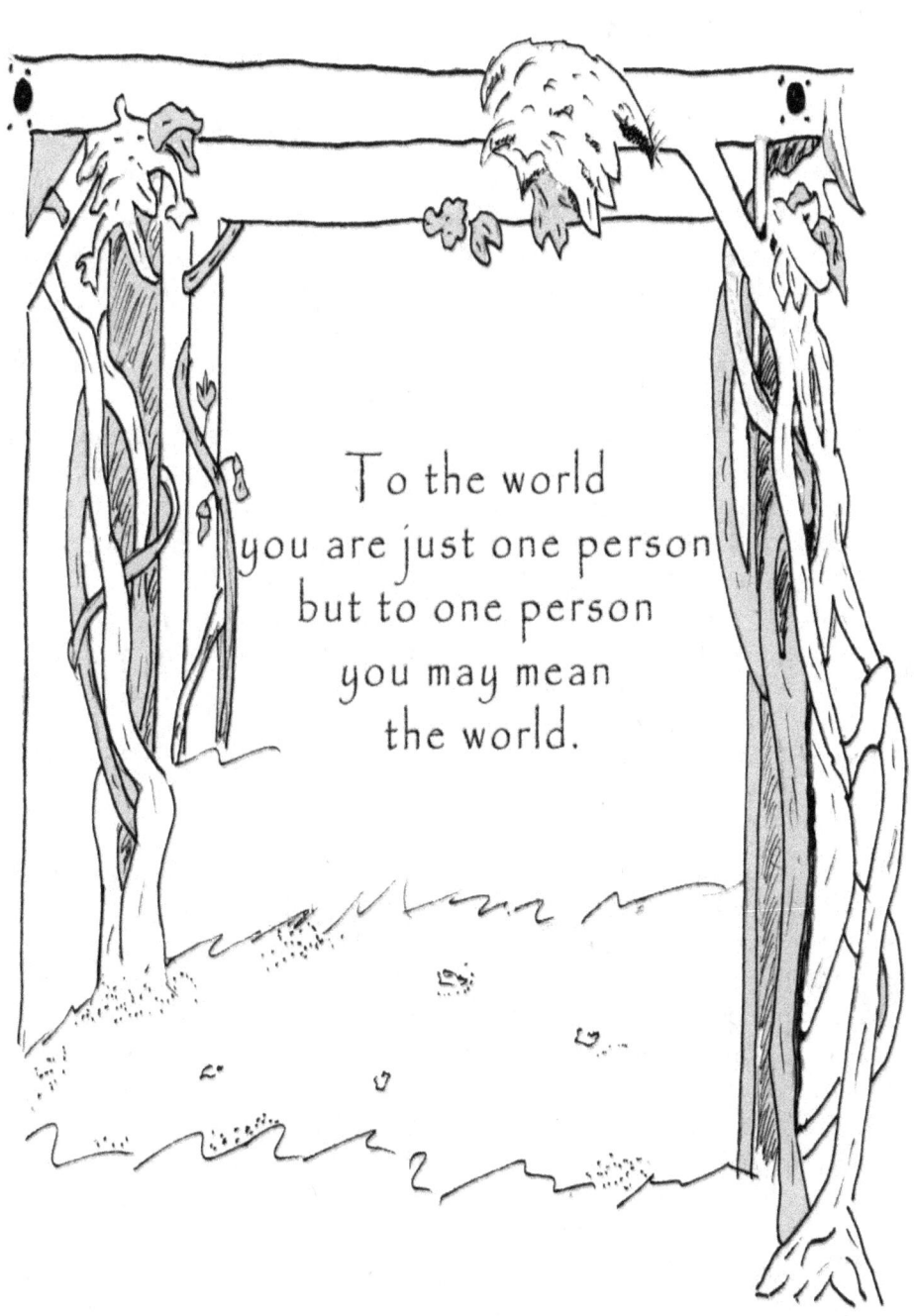

Chapter Two

My Caregiving…..The Start

When I was very young, my mother traveled for work, so I was left with others for my care. (No father in the picture and three brothers that attended military school in another state) It didn't take long to understand that I was going to be the person I turned to for entertainment, comfort, direction, and emotional support. I am not a religious person, so I tend to have a lot of conversations with the jungle of monkeys that live in my head. Early on I learned that for me there was no bonus to being sick. No one would be there to comfort me, and I would still need to do everything on my to-do list. One of my few childhood memories in grade school was a day I did in fact wake up sick. I told my mother that I didn't feel well. She said to me, "Go to school. You will feel better when you get there." I did feel better, but that was after I threw up in the hall on the way to the lunchroom. So, I guess as far as my health goes, I can credit my mother with whatever genetics she passed on as well as the "just do it anyway" attitude. Also, a bonus to my mother's empathy or lack of was that I left grade school with perfect attendance!

It was in Junior High that I first started taking care of my mother. Not in any major capacity, but assisting her and experiencing the emotions stemming from a mother that was ill. She had contracted existential pneumonia and was in pretty rough shape. This is pneumonia on the outside rather than inside the lungs. She could barely walk but as she was in a commission-based job, she needed to keep working. Just do it anyway attitude. I would help her out to her car, her boss would help her from her car up to her office, and then in the evening, the procedure was reversed. Over the years she would have several bouts of bronchitis, sinus surgeries, two hip replacements, one shoulder replacement, gastric bypass, tummy tuck, and an emergency herniated bowel surgery. She also had A-fib, microvascular disease, arthritis, inability to balance, AMD, and severe pain in one knee and one shoulder. Again, please reference my previous statement about enjoying your life now as it might not be so great when you retire. A few years ago, I heard the comedian Ricky Gervais do a little routine. He said his doctor had told him if he cut out the drinking and smoking, he could add ten years to his life. He replied, "Yeah, but those are the last ten. I don't even want those!" Really funny but also a bit of reality. Anyway...

Honestly, I don't remember specifically the emotions I had regarding my mother's health issues when I was young. For one thing, it was Junior High so enough said about that. The first real stressful moment that I do remember was years later in the waiting room during a hip replacement. It was supposed to be less than three hours but took close to four. I remember being so stressed and upset at the thought that even though it was a common procedure, that something could go wrong and she could die. Clearly that didn't happen, and clearly I didn't get the lesson that stress and projecting is a waste of time and mental fatigue. But good luck to you if you can keep yourself from repeatedly doing it.

The start of my mother's decline was developing a balance disorder. She would always refer to it as a feeling of constant motion. It wasn't vertigo and despite all the visits to neurologists, balance specialists, ENT, and the MRI, blood tests, medication trials, nothing helped. The doctor's best guess at a diagnosis was Microvascular disease (tiny little strokes in the brain affecting the area that controls balance). My own uneducated opinion is that the gastric bypass she had years earlier led to this issue. More on that and my mother later.

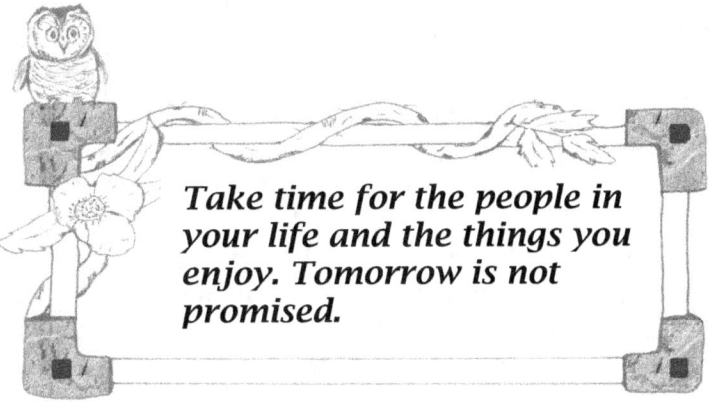

Take time for the people in your life and the things you enjoy. Tomorrow is not promised.

Things Happen For a Reason, When and How They Are Meant To

My oldest brother, Ron, was eleven years ahead of me. When he was 59, he had a quadruple bypass and two stents installed. He called it a four-banger. He was close to a visit from the Grim Reaper, but that wouldn't be his time. Mentally, I don't think he fully recovered after that operation, but that is my opinion not based on any medical diagnosis. A few years went by and after making some not so great financial decisions, he ended up losing his house he had lived in for over twenty years. He was single and faced with limited options, so his answer was to move himself into our mother's house while she was on vacation. It was meant to be temporary.

Two years younger than Ron was my brother Don. He was already living in our mother's house in the basement and had been doing so for over twenty years. Don was the picture of a heart attack waiting to happen. He lived on a daily serving from McDonalds, drank large quantities of Diet Coke, and smoked cigarettes. I would guess his weight to be around 270 pounds. One evening, Ron and Don were in the basement visiting when Ron heard a crash. Looking over towards where Don had been sitting on his bed, he now saw Don had fallen onto the floor and was wedged between his bed and a coffee table that was against the wall. He was unresponsive and despite Ron being a big guy himself, try as he might, he could not lift Don out of his entrapment. 911 was called. It took several firemen to move him and although they did try life saving measures and transported him to the hospital to be officially pronounced, I believe he was likely gone well before getting to the hospital. Ron called me after he called 911 and I rushed to the house. They were taking Don away as I was pulling up. Ron, our mother, and I drove to the hospital which was only a couple miles away. They were both praying for him, but I knew it was already a done deal. They ushered us into a tiny little room which was another obvious sign. After the "I am sorry, there was nothing we could do," we went into a room where he lay on a table. This was my first experience seeing someone 'freshly" dead. My grandmother had died several years before, and I did view her in the casket fully adorned with clown make-up. The rest of our family arrived at the hospital, and everyone cried and hugged as you would expect. I just kept thinking how strange it was to see him dead and how final that was. Clearly, I knew he was a large guy, but he seemed so much larger to me laid out on the table. It is also interesting to witness how each person deals with death so differently. For me, it seems surreal that someone just isn't on the planet anymore. Time never really lessens those thoughts although the emotions surrounding the reality of the loved one gone tend to decrease in frequency and intensity. An autopsy was done, and the cause of death was listed as Occlusive Coronary Artery Disease. Not a big surprise.

Ron and Don were best friends so Don's death was devastating for Ron. He was quite mad, convinced that Don had "left" on purpose. I suppose in some ways he did because he was a smart guy, and he knew that the way he was treating his body/health would reward him with a short life span. Mom and Ron tried numerous times to get him to stop smoking and/or eat better. My feelings are that everyone gets to drive their own car. Maybe he had no interest in living to his not so golden years. Anyway, I firmly believe that Don would not have been able to handle what was to come for Ron or our mother. This also brings up the question, is the unexpected death of someone better or worse than a slow decline?

At his graveside I said to the family, "Be sure to live your life to the fullest and leave nothing unsaid or no "bad blood" with those you love as you never know what the future holds for you or your loved one." Also, as I will mention later, even if you have time with your loved one at the end, they may not be in a mental state to understand or discuss anything with you.

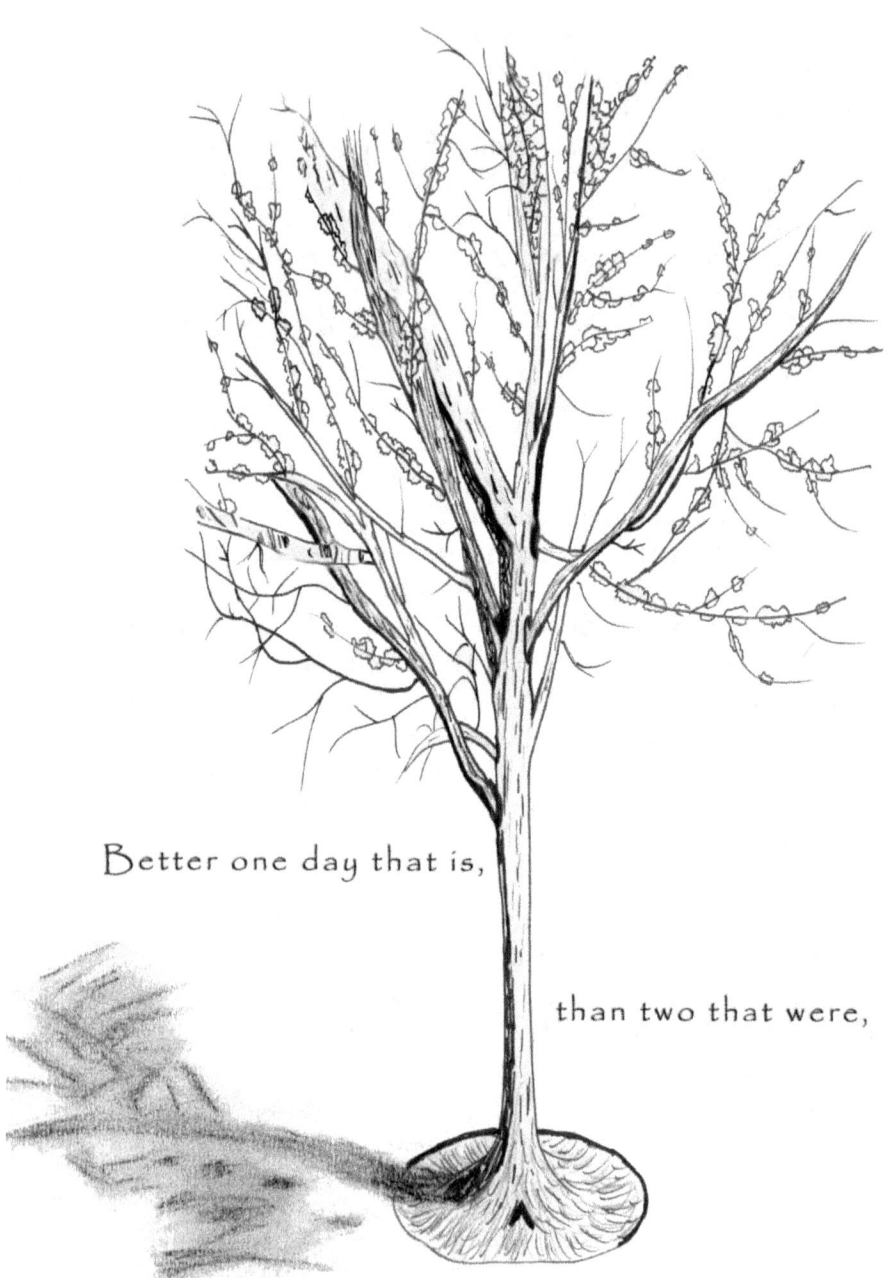

Better one day that is,

than two that were,

or three that will never be.....

Understanding the Medical Industry
Ask Questions

One day Ron had me look at a patch of skin on his back that was kind of dry and scaly. It didn't look like a big deal; I suggested a couple of different ointments. When it didn't go away, he went to a dermatologist. I questioned him after his return. What was it? His answer: "I don't know. I didn't ask." Really? He said the doctor prescribed a strong antibiotic cream. I suggested that it might be a good idea to know what was growing on him and why. Subsequent calls revealed that it was Sarcoidosis.

Although he had no interest in doing research, I on the other hand jumped on it. Sarcoidosis is a disease involving abnormal collection of inflammatory cells that form lumps known as granulomas. The disease usually begins in the lungs, skin, or lymph nodes. The cause is unknown. Apparently, the professionals don't become alarmed or interested unless it is detected in the blood. The professionals said his blood was negative for Sarcoidosis. Interesting…..

I was more concerned about it than he was. He was fine with his cream although it didn't ever completely go away. The medical professionals give you minimal if any information and if you don't ask, they won't tell. I found if you ask enough questions, you can really piss doctors off. Whether it is in regard to your own health or the person you are taking care of, you must ask questions. Well, I guess you don't have to. You can blindly take or dole out whatever medication is prescribed; you can have or take your loved one for whatever surgery or procedure is suggested. And then, you can sit back and see what happens next, what drug, procedure, or what surgery will be suggested next and next and next.

If you are open to this concept of being informed, there is a part B. You must also research. Research will assist you in asking the right questions. Much has been said about the misinformation on the internet. You will find that like any topic even non-medical ones, you can find just about any take on your subject. Many sites you will notice have the exact same wording. If you search a broad topic, you will get an enormous amount of potential information to sift through. The more specific you get or perhaps the rarer the issue, mostly what you will find will be clinical papers or nothing at all. Unfortunately, unless you are of that mind set, clinical papers are very challenging to read. I usually scrolled down to the end to see if it had any value for me, or if I could understand the summary.

No one is going to award you a degree for all your new knowledge, but it can put you in the driver's seat with respect to the medical industry. Maybe that drug isn't needed. Maybe the new drug is causing other problems. Maybe that procedure will do more harm in the long run, are there alternatives? Consider physical therapy, weight loss, changing diet, eliminating something, adding something. You can spend an enormous amount of time researching, and the situation may warrant that amount of time. You can also devote a small amount of time that it takes to be informed, which might just save you and your "patient" lots of time and frustration in the future.

Do I have a negative perception of the medical industry? Yes. I had this perception prior to being immersed in it with my family. Some of it comes from reading books, some from observation of others and their experiences, and some from eighteen years spent in the healthcare field, not as a clinician but as a medical recruiter. My job was to find sales professionals for medical and pharmaceutical companies. When I started an assignment, although I didn't have to, I liked to do a little research. I can't help it; it's just who I am. I wanted to know about the company, product, competitors, etc. Some assignments were fun, straight forward, even interesting. Some were not. Many times, I couldn't help but think, why would someone risk taking that drug or doing that procedure? Even though I thought the product or procedure very unnecessary in the world, my job required a certain amount of "selling" to get the candidate to change jobs. You might be able to see my problem; how do I sell someone on something I don't believe in? Another factor was the salaries/commissions that many sales representatives made. It varied anywhere from a very respectable living to living large. Some of these products were not any better than what was already available for cheap but because it was the new hot item, it was going to be marketed heavily and of course be more expensive. So, when you are prescribed a drug or a procedure is suggested, is it the best for you or is it the hot new item? Orthopedics has been a hot bed for many years. Many doctors/surgeons have their own companies or vested interest in the products they use to "repair" you. And even if the doctor didn't have his/her hand in the cookie jar, the hospital likely negotiated the best deal for its bottom line. Is that really the best "part" they are going to put in your body or the one they got the best deal on? Is the procedure really going to be a long-term benefit to you without repercussions or is it a money maker for the hospital? A saying you may have heard before: "It is all about the money." Sorry to say, that sums up most of the world but certainly applies to the medical industry. There are countless books written pro and con on the medical industry. One I read is, **"An American Sickness, How Healthcare Became Big Business And How You Can Take It Back"** by Elisabeth Rosenthal. She does a great job of explaining how the industry works. However, I don't think we will be taking it back any time soon if ever. Like a lot of topics in America these days, it has as I like to say, gone to hell in a handbag.

There are repercussions from medical decisions made for yourself and your loved ones. It is hard to consider everything. In her book, **"Knocking on Heaven's Door"** Katy Butler describes how her family agreed to put a pacemaker in her dad being advised of its necessity. Later when the rest of him had really gone south, the pacemaker kept right on ticking for him. Shutting it off was not an option, so the family and unfortunately the dad had to ride it out. It is a great book and just one example of the need to analyze medical decisions thoroughly, maybe life saving measures are not the right choice.

My partner was told she had to have her gall bladder out. No options were mentioned. Also, no long-term effects were mentioned. So, for the rest of her life, she had difficulty eating fats even the good-for-you-kind, then spent several years suffering with pancreatitis. How different would life have been if gall bladder health had been addressed rather than the gall bladder removed? My mother had a gastric bypass, then never absorbed nutrients properly again, at minimum being chronically anemic the remainder of her life.

The medical industry has a term called Informed Consent. In the American Medical Association's code of ethics, it states that "informed consent to medical treatment is fundamental in both ethics and law. Patients have the right to receive information and ask questions about recommended treatments so that they can make well-considered decisions about care." Despite it being a basic patient right, often no real discussions take place. (Other than to make sure your insurance will cover it!)

It isn't all bad and thank goodness doctors/surgeons are there when we really need them. Although I don't go to doctors, I had a ladder "incident" and needed them to stitch my face. Very happy that I had access to that service, and they did a fabulous job. I just think we have put too much blind faith in doctors and the industry and need to take charge of our own temples and if need be, our own "ending."

Clearly, urgent care is a different scenario than what I am discussing. If you are having a heart attack or stroke, there is no time for research or for considering alternatives. Elective surgical procedures, chronic issues, and long-term medicating I feel would benefit from extra research and thought before moving forward. This is my perspective. I don't want to discourage you from seeking professional diagnosis or help, just encouraging extra thought.

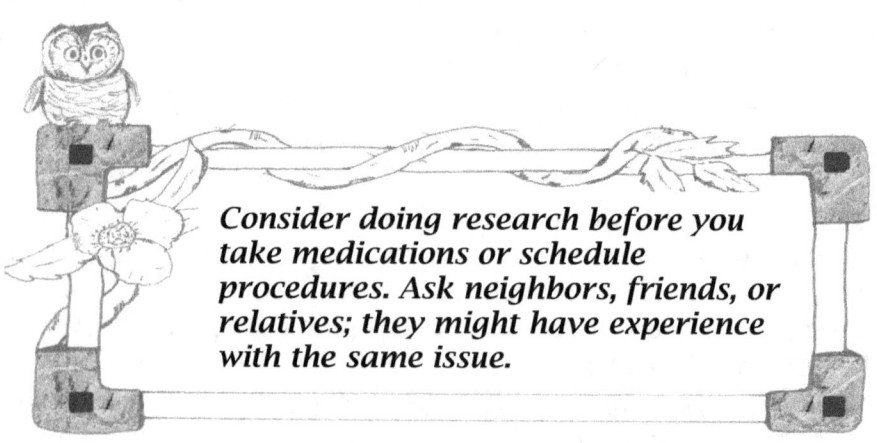

Consider doing research before you take medications or schedule procedures. Ask neighbors, friends, or relatives; they might have experience with the same issue.

More Health Concerns for Ron

Sometimes you can see a person from a different perspective than they see themselves. Ron was having trouble breathing, winded at very simple tasks. In addition, he complained of not really pain but an uncomfortable feeling right under his breastbone. I suggested that he see a doctor. As he didn't have insurance, he went to a local clinic for testing. It had been about six years since his "four-banger," so I was concerned that he had a blockage again. Everyone knows that heart patients usually require a new eating or exercise routine. Not Ron. I have never run across anyone more obsessed with their food. He could reference specifics about foods or restaurants that he experienced as a young child. Going to a restaurant with him was truly an experience. Everything had to be exactly the way he remembered and liked it. Expecting him to not heap the potato with enormous quantities of butter and sour cream was a pipe dream. Needless to say, in addition to a family history of high cholesterol and heart issues, his diet did nothing to extend his life.

Tests were done.

A Tale of Two Patients

Years earlier, my mother had a building built next to her house to accommodate her business. I ended up working for her in that business which allowed me to be with her daily. Her balance issue had become very challenging for her. She tried all the professionals' suggestions but to no avail. In her words, she said it "felt like she was in constant motion." If you tried to call it dizzy or vertigo, she would say that was incorrect. None the less, it made life difficult. She had a hard time with anything that required hand eye coordination. This issue had been developing for about ten years, so by the time she was in her 80's her age had also contributed to her mobility and coordination challenge. In addition to the balance issue, she also began having difficulty getting up from a sitting position. Seeing her struggle, I saw the need for retrofitting her house and office for safety concerns. These changes were done over several years, and I will discuss some of them in the next chapter and others later as I utilized them. Obviously, everyone will have different issues and different environments but much of what is available is the same.

Over the years, my mother had several medical issues and procedures, most of which I either took her to or helped her rehab from. It doesn't seem like a lot until you start a list. In no order: two hip replacements, shoulder replacement, sinus surgeries, cataract surgery, Afib (cardio revascularization), Synvisc injections, AMD (eye injections), LRTI (Thumb surgery), shingles, microvascular disease, tummy tuck, Gastric bypass, herniated bowel surgery, numerous MRI's, CT's, Pneumonia, Cdiff, Etc, Etc. Surely, I have forgotten a few things, but I think the picture is clear. It is amazing what the body will power through. Most of what I want to convey in this book stems from my experience during the last three years of her life. I do however want to mention a few things about some of the previous surgeries.

My mother was a very attractive lady. Beginning in the 1960's she worked in male dominated industries and made it a point to always look like a million dollars. Fit, stylish, and ready to take on whatever was dished out. Her accomplishments were impressive. On the flip side of that positiveness was the constant struggle with weight. Over her lifetime, she left no diet untried, joined all the groups and eating plans, read all the books, drank all the shakes and meal replacements, even went for a month to a health retreat in southern Utah. In her late 70's she underwent what I like to call the stupid surgery. A completely asinine risky procedure known as the Tummy Tuck. But it was her body and certainly not up to me, so she had it done, and I helped her recoup from it. The incisions needed draining. Grrrr. And no, it didn't help a damn thing.

Much earlier, while in her 50's, she had put on a fair bit of weight and in the pursuit and quest for the perfect image, opted for a surgery, a gastric bypass. We were not really relating well at that time, so I didn't help her recoup with this one, although I believe in the end, I did. It is my opinion that all surgeries carry risk and if the surgery is unnecessary as this procedure was, the benefits do not outweigh the potential negative outcomes. Other than the typical before surgery disclaimers that they give for all procedures, they don't explain one big issue with this procedure and to be fair, I doubt anyone wanting the procedure would listen. Gastric bypass causes malabsorption and nutrient deficiencies. In addition to this, the duodenum, a major area of nutrient absorption within the intestinal tract, may be bypassed depending on the type of procedure performed, further contributing to nutrient deficiencies. It is my completely unprofessional opinion that years of low iron and lack of B12 absorption either contributed to or caused the microvascular/balance issues later in life. She also needed several rounds of iron shots over the years. If that wasn't enough of a side effect, the procedure created an area, or pocket if you will, that allowed the bowel to get tangled requiring an emergency Volvulus surgery (herniated bowel). This happened about three years prior to her death. It was her final surgery and one that she never really recovered from.

Life is not how well you execuite plan A

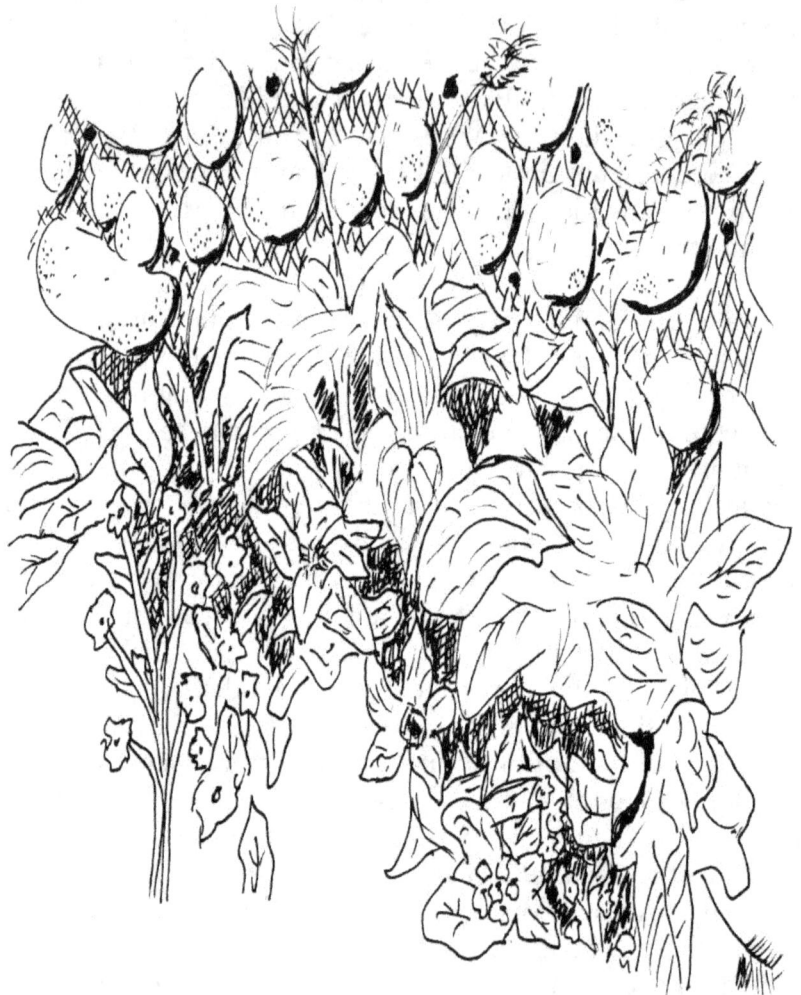

It is how well you adjust to Plan B

Chapter Three

Mobility Aids

Safety 1st!
There are some easy changes you can make to help mobility be a little safer around the house that won't cost you a dime. Moving clutter, extra furniture, and of course removing the dreaded throw rugs. These things are easy to negotiate for younger agile folks but not for those with challenges. Also, those with vision problems like AMD or glaucoma have difficulty distinguishing between surface transitions. For instance, carpet to linoleum or a level surface to a step up or down. You want to make sure these transitions are very "seeable."

The first alteration I did was to add grab bars. These are available in various colors and sizes. I installed them in the shower, by the toilet (side wall and wall in front), and the top of the stairs as once my mother made it to the top, the railing had ended and there was nothing but flat wall to grab at. Her staircase from ground floor to the upstairs bedrooms had never had an outside railing so a wooden banister was added there and metal railings on both buildings' entrances. Later as stairs were more of a herculean feat, she would pull herself up, grabbing and pulling on both rails. That was no problem. Later, when her left arm became basically useless, she would pull by the outside rail only. As it was wooden, I watched it get more and more rickety as time went on. In retrospect, I would have had that installed more structurally sound than what companies might normally do for a staircase.

A note here regarding stairs: We did consider a stair lift. We decided against it initially and after subsequent events that I will cover later, it wasn't a great option for us. They are also $4000+ and of course like anything else you might need, not covered by Medicare. If you have the room and money, you can also have a lift or elevator installed.

On the outside stairs I purchased different ramps based on the height/rise needed. If you have one or maybe two stairs, an adjustable pair like the ones pictured below are a great option. In addition to being relatively inexpensive, they are transportable. If you need to take your person to someone's house, chances are they are going to have stairs that you will need to transverse. Ramps are available in all different shapes and sizes; these handle regular wheelchairs or transport chairs well. You can find them from multiple sources. Nearly all the "aids" I purchased came from Amazon.

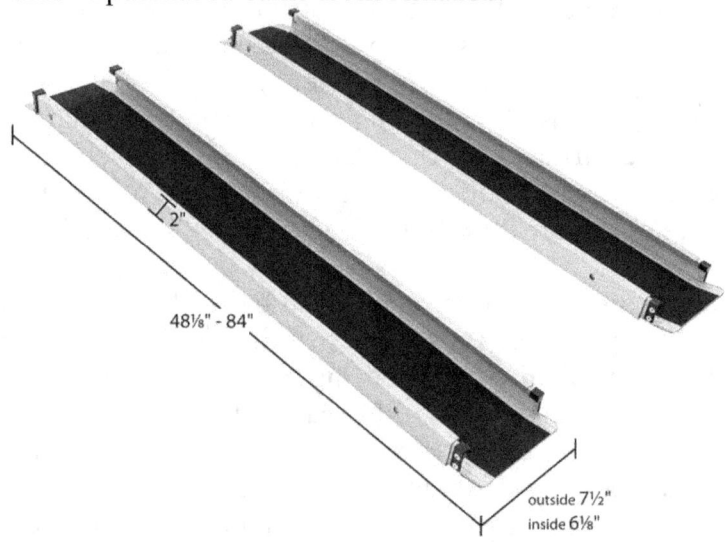

Another entrance I needed to tackle had five stairs, so ramps like the ones above are not appropriate. If money is no option, then call a handy person and have a custom ramp built for your situation. Medicare does not pay for ramps. However, many states offer Medicaid Waivers which pay for the cost of ramps, as they are considered home modifications or environmental adaptations and help to prevent / and or delay unnecessary nursing home placements, saving the state money. You would need to qualify for Medicaid for these benefits (not Medicare). Also, it is my understanding that Habitat for Humanity has a program for low-income seniors for building ramps.
https://www.habitat.org/volunteer/near-you/find-your-local-habitat
The ADA guidelines for ramps state that they should be 36" wide, handrails on both sides should be at 34-38", and the length depends on

the amount of height or rise you need. As an example, 30" would require a 30-foot ramp. I didn't do that. Also, according to the ADA if you have to have a turn, the landing should be 5' x 5'. Although I had about a 30" rise, I didn't have 30 feet without going over the lawn or driveway, so I just did what worked. I purchased a kit on Amazon that had the metal hardware. I purchased an 8' sheet of ¾" plywood from the hardware store and had them cut to it to 36" width and then in half so I had two pieces 4' x 36". Using a drill, screwdriver, and a socket wrench, I put it all together and put it in place. In short order, I learned that it wasn't going to work with just 8 feet of ramp. There was a scary moment for me at the top when I thought we might both be headed backwards down the ramp, it was just a bit too steep. Yikes! A ramp kit didn't come any longer, so I decided to buy another 8-foot kit. I had to drill some holes in the metal to make it possible to add a four-foot section, but it worked, and 12 feet worked fine for me. Depending on your physical capabilities, you may find that you may have no choice but to have someone build you a custom version. My ramp is pictured here. Also note that in addition to being less than the recommended length, I did not put handrails. My mother was never going to use the wheelchair on her own and I didn't feel like I needed them. I will tell you though that some older visitors were a little scared of walking the ramp. Also, in my situation, we could still walk up the stairs on the left side of the ramp.

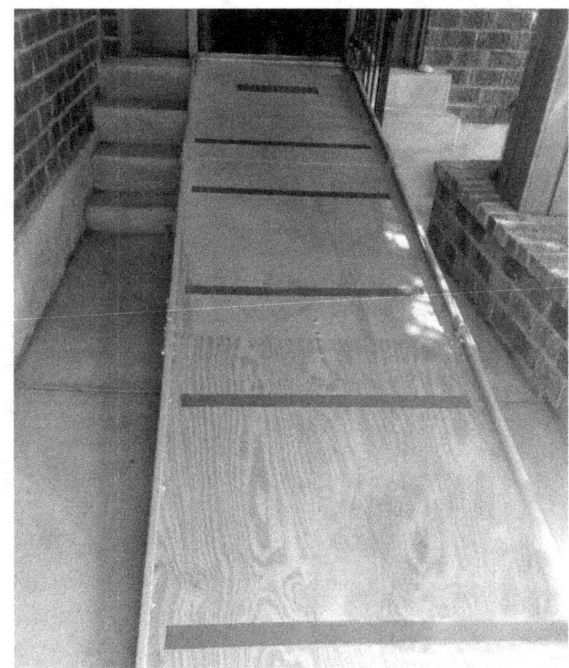

Walkers-Rollators-Canes and Such

Over the course of taking care of someone their abilities and needs change, so it is likely that you will find yourself with an array of different walking aids.

I don't know why but it seems the dreaded cane is met with a fair amount of resistance. Maybe it is a symbol of old age or an admission that help is needed, but my mother wouldn't have anything to do with it initially. She had a cane that she had utilized previously when rehabbing from a hip replacement, but I guess that was different.

Rollators:

I believe the rollator was the first device we purchased. These come in all colors and prices. Ours was basic like the one on the left, under $100.

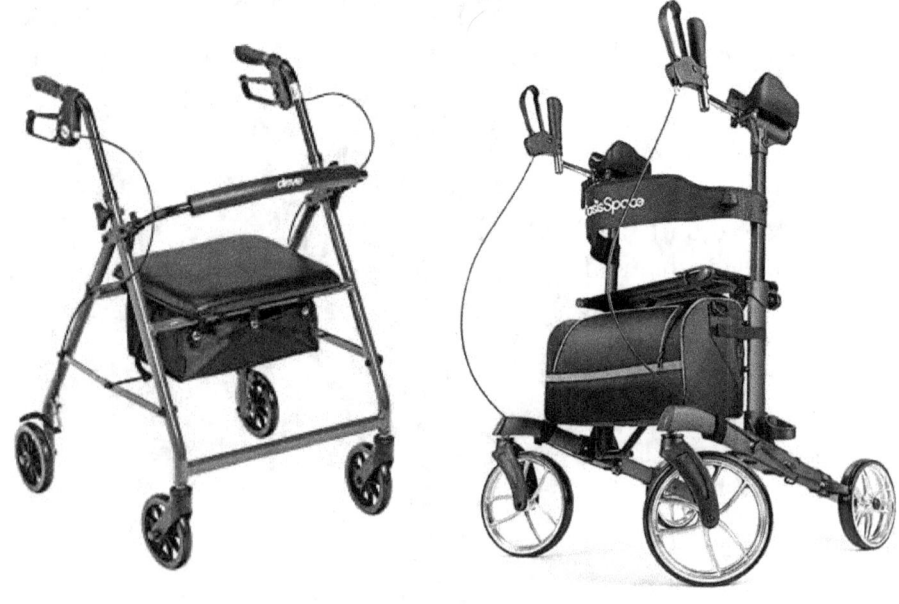

Rollators can have baskets, larger wheels, more substantial frames, seats, arm rests that are adjustable, and more. The nice part about these as opposed to a walker is that they do have the ability to sit. If that is a feature you need, make sure to check the seat height before you purchase as some are a bit low and will be a challenge for your person to get up from. They all have brakes, are light weight, and fold up making it easy to toss in the car. You can push the person as they sit on it but……Once I ignored my intuition and let my mother walk with it to the neighbors for book club night. Of course, she was too tired to walk back so she sat, and I pushed. It was going well until I hit a crack in the sidewalk. Not sure how she wasn't dumped on the ground but for me that put an end to using the rollator in that manner.

Walkers:

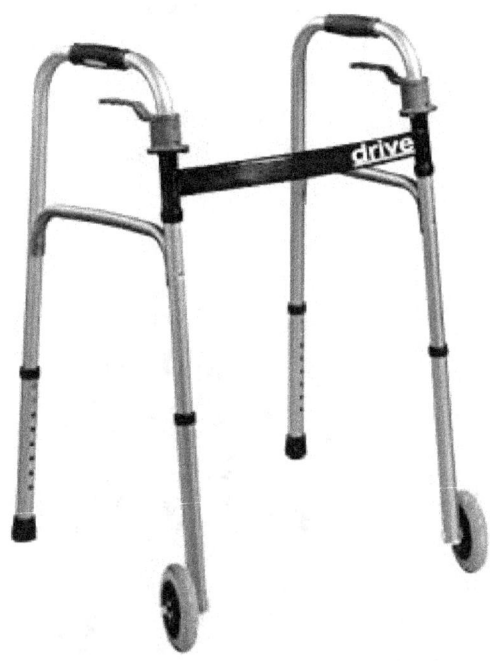

Just like the rollator, walkers can certainly be used when you need to go out in public. If you need the person to go a little slower, these are a good option. We had one for inside the house which of course we retrofitted with the obligatory tennis balls. The tennis balls are placed on the legs without wheels so that it can roll across the carpet or wood floor easier. These also come without wheels so that the person has to pick it up, move it forward, and walk into it. That is how the walker should work regardless of the style, but good luck getting your person to do it correctly. The tendency is for them to push it out in front with arms extended like they are racing a shopping cart to a blue light special. In addition to going too fast, it causes them to be hunched over rather than standing up straight. Make sure the walker is set at the right height. If they are standing by the walker with arms hanging down, the handles should be at the same level as their wrists. These also fold up for easy storage or transport.

Wheelchairs/Transport Chairs

There came a point where walking for any distance was too difficult so a walker or rollator would not do. Wheelchairs can be very basic, and they can be very deluxe and expensive (ranging from $100 to $3000). I chose a basic model wheelchair. It needed to be collapsible and not overly heavy so I could toss it in the back of the car when we went places. Another option is a transport chair. They have all four wheels small rather than the two big wheels that allow the person to roll themselves. If you are always going to push, the transport chair might be your better choice as it is lighter. Here are a couple of tips on wheelchair operation. The first one, when I realized how difficult I was making it for myself, I was a little embarrassed. The footrests need to move out of the way when you are getting close to the car or perhaps pulling your person up to a table. I was taking them off. @%X*! They happen to easily swing back towards the big wheel as the one in the picture below.

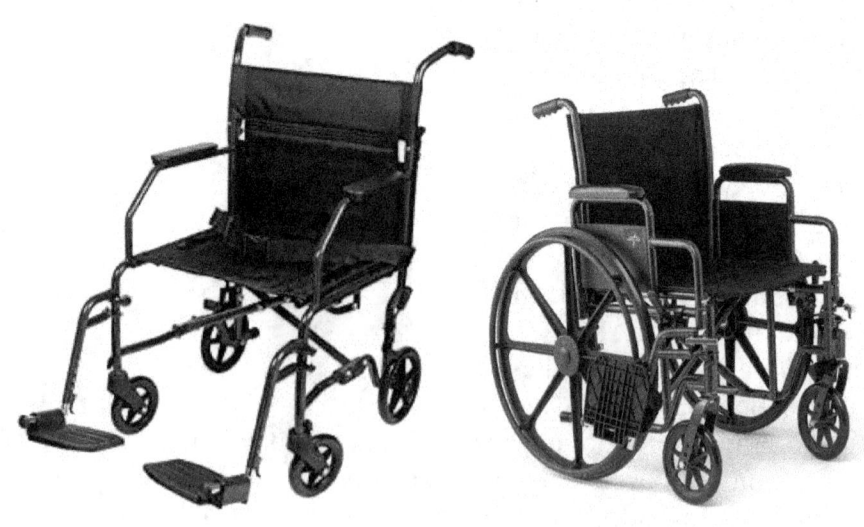

The second tip is for when you need to go over a threshold or small step. As you are pushing the chair, there are two bars at the bottom, one on each side. Put your foot on one, push down as you pull back on the handles. Kind of like "popping a wheely." The chair moves back fairly easy even with a heavy occupant.

I had a cheap model wheelchair that I could easily lift in and out of the car. When I started taking my mother for a neighborhood stroll, I found it to be a bit rickety. Through a community listing I was able to find a barely used wheelchair for $200 that was originally about a $3000 model. It was able to tilt back which made going down the ramp seem less scary and it had much better suspension so the sidewalk strolls didn't seem quite so bumpy.

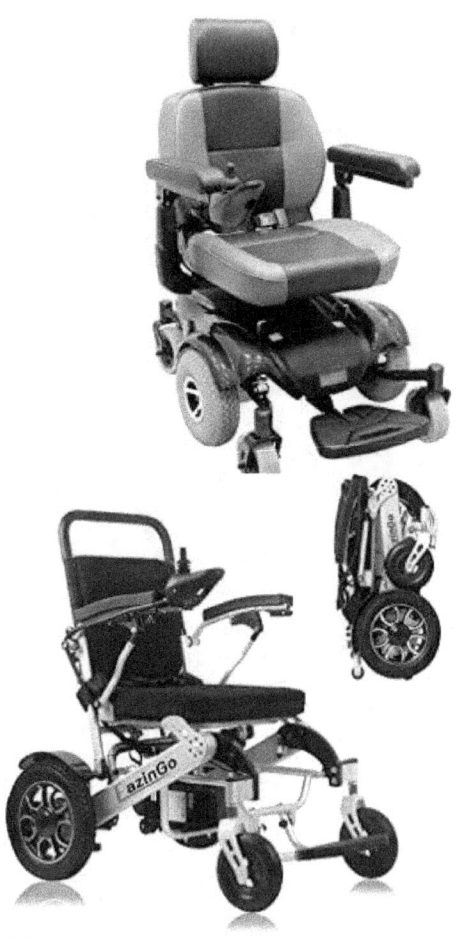

Wheelchairs can be obtained through online sources such as Amazon, through local medical supply companies, and secondary sources such as thrift stores and local online community listings. Wheelchairs are considered DME or Durable Medical Equipment. Depending on your insurance and your doctor's recommendation, you may be able to obtain products "rented" to you with a co-pay.

Canes

Television is such a big part of life for seniors and if you have watched it for more than just a casual amount of time, then you are aware of the allure of marketing. Yes, among other things, we needed a HurryCane. We had two colors. Their pitch, in addition to the user having the freedom of mobility, (apparently with it, they could now go anywhere!), it could stand on its own. How clever is that? It works. Until they use it for awhile and wear out the little pads unevenly, then it falls on the floor like other canes. But they are stylish. Canes are a great help in the beginning if your person is still ambulatory.

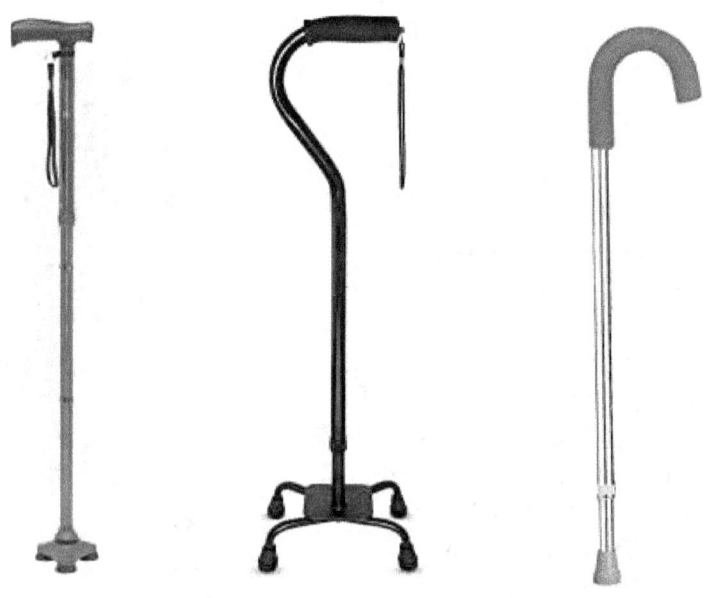

Chairs

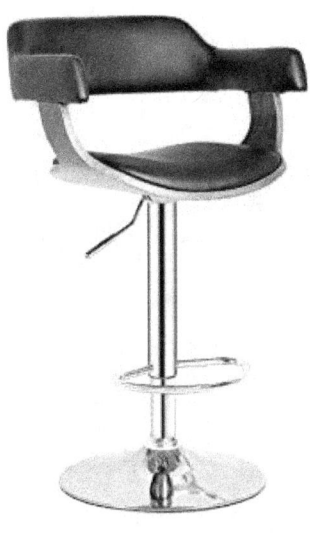

Since in my mother's situation chairs and getting out of them were an issue, I tried to find chairs that had arms and a seat that was a bit higher than normal. Although fluffy puffy chairs are comfy, they are challenging to get out of. They do make chairs that have an auto lift feature, but they are bulky and would not have been to my patient's taste!

The breakfast bar had regular wooden bar stools that did not hold up to daily stress particularly the backs. They became unstable in a very short time. I found a padded bar stool with arms that had adjustable height as well as a swivel. It didn't match a thing but made it easier to get on and off.

It was such a challenge to go places. I tried my best to make sure my mother sat in chairs that I could help her get out of but sometimes it was a struggle. The care centers use a belt that they put around the person and pull them up standing face to face. As my mother had a severe balance issue, standing right in front of her wasn't an option. In addition, her shoulder/arm became so painful for her, she didn't want that touched. I ended up always getting her up from the side which I became very good at but really isn't the safest method to not injure the caregiver.

Unfortunately, going places where she couldn't stay in the wheelchair became just too difficult. In addition to chairs being a challenge to get up from, toilets were an issue.

Bathrooms

Early on I strategically installed multiple handrails in the bathrooms. At a certain point the toilet was too low for ease of sitting or getting back up. I tried all the different seat risers. They are different depending on the shape of your toilet, but they all work ok to some degree. You will have to continue to ensure that the connections are tight because the pressure from usage loosens the bolts on a regular basis. Depending on the space you have on the sides of the toilet, you can utilize ones that have handrails. Also, if you have a portable potty, sometimes referred to as a bedside potty (pictured to the right) and don't need it bedside yet, remove the catch bucket and it can be placed over the toilet rather than attaching a riser.

Another option is to change out the toilet for an ADA approved one. They are typically around 17" from floor to seat which is a couple of inches taller than most. I happened to have found a commercial one that was 18". It does make it easier to stand up from if getting up is an issue. It also makes it very challenging for kids to use if that is a consideration for you. If the floor in the bathroom is not carpeted, it can be a slick surface to stand up from the toilet. I secured a rubber anti-fatigue mat to the floor which allowed for some extra traction.

Showers/Baths

Bathtubs become a scary place for seniors or those with disabilities. Having an actual bath is very challenging and most opt for quick showers. And those showers are not wanted very often! Stepping into a regular bathtub can be very spooky if you are already unsteady on your feet, plus you are stepping onto a slick surface then adding water, so it is no easy feat. To help ensure a safe experience, there should be one or more bars mounted on the wall, perhaps on both the outside wall and inside wall. Add bath grip-stickers or a non-slip floor mat. A shower chair maybe necessary if standing is a challenge.

In my case we had a 4" rise to enter the shower. That doesn't seem like much but that even became an issue. I found a shower chair that worked quite well. It was a bench shape, a person sitting on one side of the bench could raise or have their feet raised and be pushed to the other side of the bench and into the shower. Reverse the process when done.

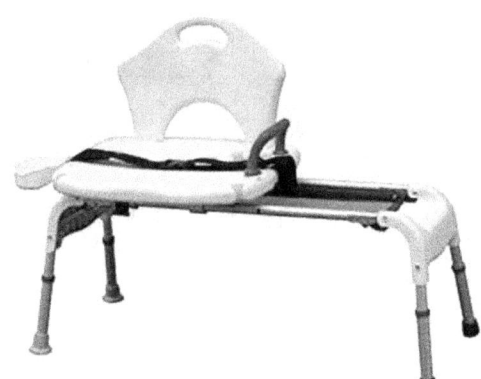

This type of shower bench is also available with a chair that swivels which might be convenient depending on your situation. This one is a little over $100. Swiveled versions are closer to $300.

There is also one available that has a removable section in the center of the seat to give better access for cleaning. This bench can work with a tub or shower. Even if an older person is still showering themselves, it can be a safer alternative than a chair in the tub which can be more challenging to get on and off of.

They make a substantial front handrail (pictured to the right) if your person is still getting in the tub on their own. Again, if you are on a budget, don't forget to check out second hand, thrift stores, or local internet-based sales forums for some of your mobility items.

Available at home stores or via the internet you can find a kit that will convert the tub to a "walk in" shower by cutting the tub and installing the insert shown below. It will run you $300+ and could be a great lower cost option than a full tub conversion.

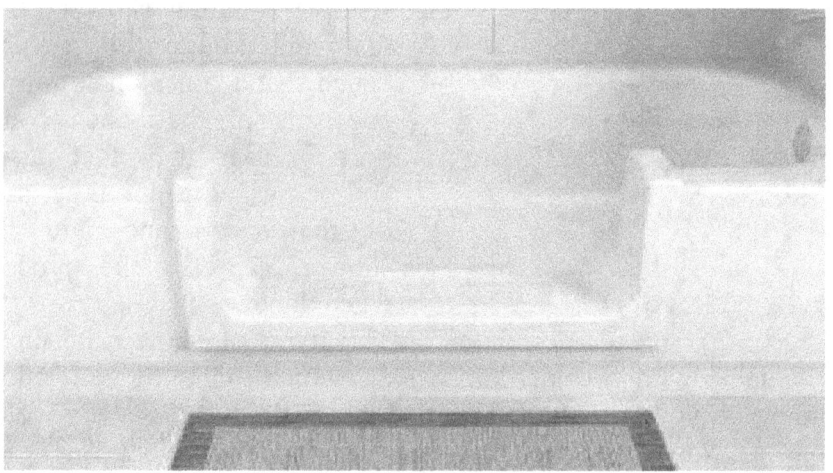

Regarding all the aids you purchase, when you no longer need them, if you have space, you may want to store them. Chances are good that you will again have a need for some of it or know someone you can pass it on to.

Vehicle Assist

If you need to help someone in and out of a car which has a little lower seat and no handle to pull up on, there is a small device that you put in the latch area of the car when the door is open and remove it after the person exits the car.

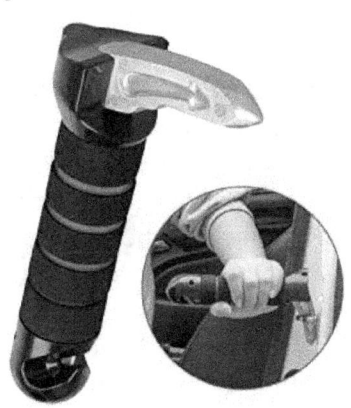

When I first started driving my mother places, I had a truck. At that time, she was able to pull herself up with the handle inside the truck, but the running board was too high of a step. I got this little step with a handle which aided in her getting the right height to pull herself in.

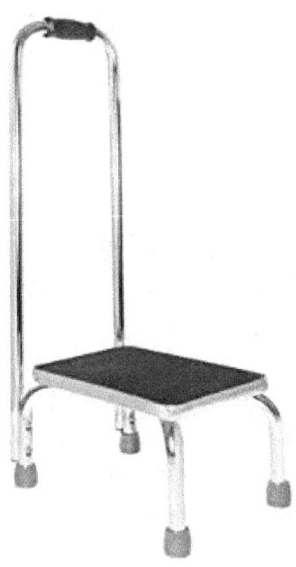

Same on the way out. Without this step, it was way too far of a drop. Later the truck was a no-go, so I got a car. A major consideration for my purchase was making sure that the seats were at a height that allowed for an easy in and out and the back area was large enough to accommodate a wheelchair.

Bed Assist

Several years prior to her needing assistance, my mother purchased a bed that was powered to move the head or feet up and down. This came in really handy during the care phase because she could sit up into a comfortable position without ten pillows propping her up. It was also a little higher than some beds making it easier for her to get off of, yet not as high as some people like their beds that appear to need a running leap or stool to get into. I installed one of these devices making it safer for my mother to steady herself to a standing position and to have something firm to hold on to while getting her walker in place. No matter where in the bed she was initially situated, she would always end up tilted towards the edge and the thought of her falling off was a real possibility. This device goes between the mattress and box springs to hold it in place. It really came in handy the last several months as she needed it to both steady her as she got on her feet and to help her get into bed and situate correctly. As with all the devices I have mentioned, there are several versions available. If you get a device like this, make sure to measure the distance you need from the box springs to the floor as there is only so much adjustment possible.

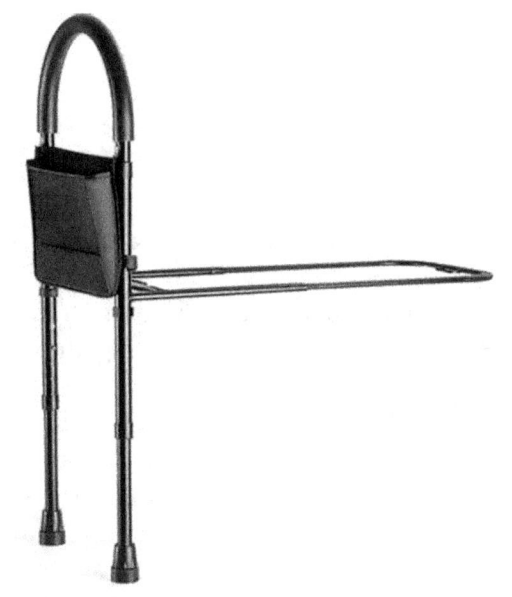

Vision Assistance

Losing eyesight is not a fun time. My mother had AMD, Age Related Macular Degeneration. This results in the loss of seeing in the center vision of your eye. Glaucoma results in the outer vision being lost. Of course, there are many other reasons for the loss of sight other than age related changes. Vision loss can be a big change of life for the person as well as those around them. I have worn contacts since I was ten and I currently have a pair of reading glasses in every room, in the car, in the garage, the shed, etc. That hassle is dwarfed by serious vision loss.

For my mother the start of the obvious vision loss was that on more than one occasion she whacked the mirror on the side of the garage when backing her car out. Then came a fender bender. She finally admitted that she was scared to drive. That did not mean she wanted to part with her Cadillac convertible. This is a tough subject for most seniors and those wanting to keep them safe. The loss of independence by not being able to drive is difficult. It didn't matter that I was willing to drive her anywhere. She had been a goer all her life. Shopping, errands, plays, concerts, church, movies, restaurants, and much more. Not to be able to jump in her car and go was, I think, a major turning point in her spirit.

The other major activity that was adversely affected was reading. She was an avid reader of books, daily reader of the local paper and Wall Street Journal. We transferred the Journal to her computer. Within your computer settings you can increase the font size for all data quite a bit. That even became a challenge as again the center of vision is impaired. We tried several hand-held or full-page magnifiers, but nothing seemed to help much.

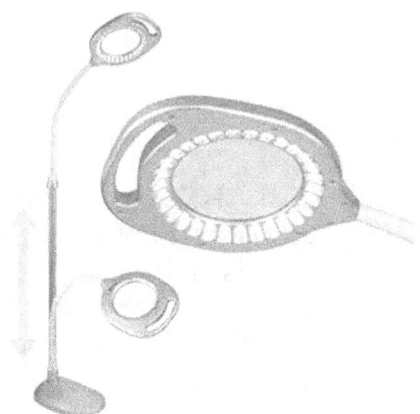

If someone was still active with crafts and such, there are several floor model magnifiers that include a light which can be handy for those of us that haven't lost all vision!

Once reading on her own was too difficult, I got an Audible account for a Fire tablet and hooked it up to auxiliary speakers, so it was easier to hear. That worked well until comprehension became an issue. Not only were the novels difficult to follow, but the last several months even the news programs on TV didn't always make sense to her.

Injections for Age Related Macular Degeneration
There are two forms of AMD, dry and wet. There is no treatment for dry other than the suggested vitamins. At the time (2015) the suggestion for my mother's wet version was injections of bevacizumab. This was an "off label" use. Bevacizumab is approved to treat metastatic colorectal cancer. There are enormous amounts of drugs that are used "off label." This means that the FDA has not approved it for the new application that the doctors are prescribing it for. It may in fact be effective for treating the new condition that it is being used for, but it has not gone through the clinical trial/approval process. Aside from all that, she had the injections for a couple of years, but the eyesight continued to decline and at a certain point the Ophthalmologist said it would be of no use to continue the injections. The doctor gave us a letter stating that she was legally blind. The Social Security Administration does offer assistance for the blind. Rather than Social Security income it is SSI or Supplemental Security Income. They do a means test with this supplement so if you are already receiving a large monthly Social Security Benefit, you may not qualify.   https://www.ssa.gov/benefits/ssi

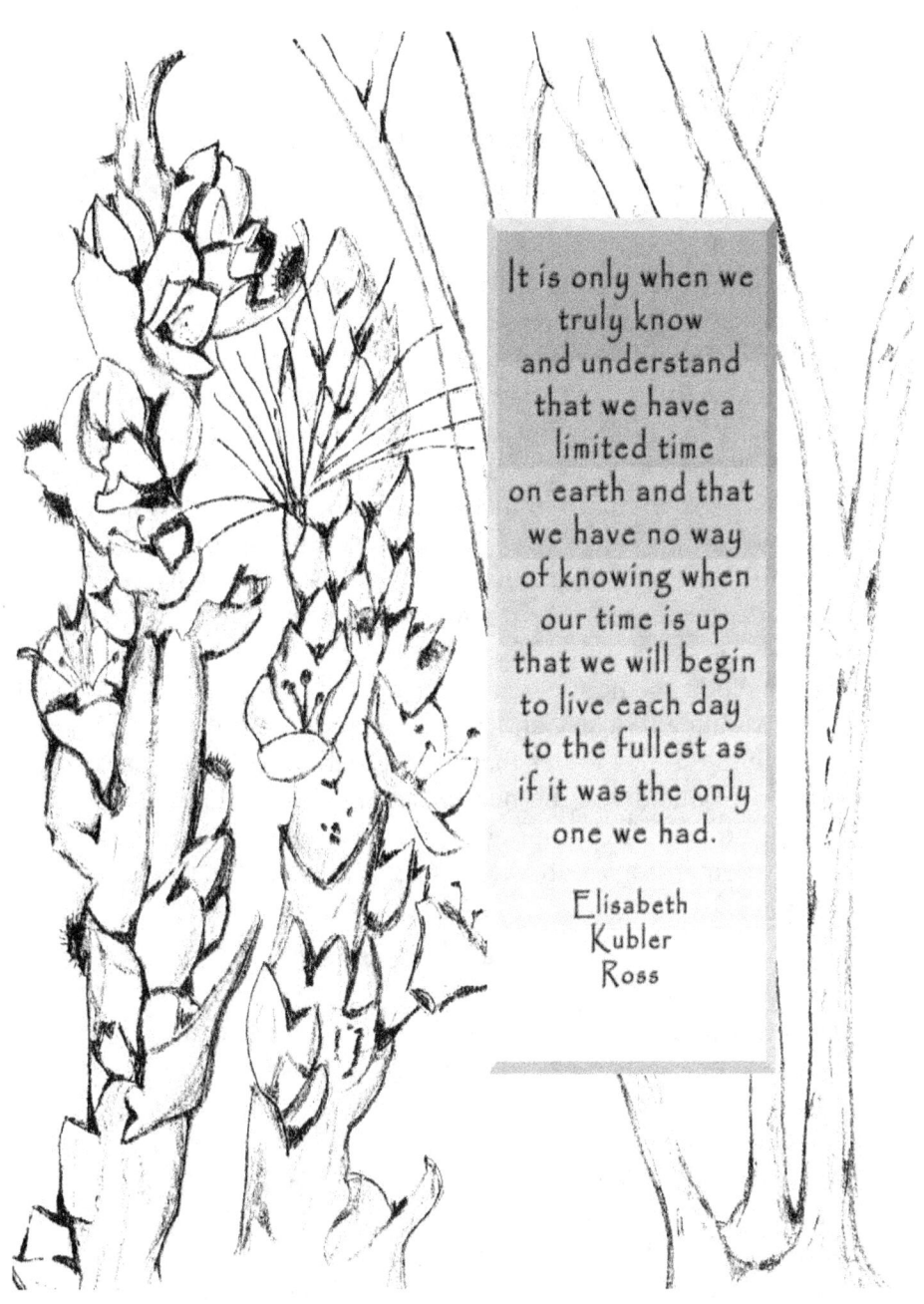

Chapter Four

Back To Ron..
The Diagnosis before the Diagnosis

Blood tests for Ron showed that he had high C Reactive Protein and Triglycerides. That led to a Nuclear Cardiac Test or Pet Scan. Apparently, the valve that had two stents inserted six years prior had scar tissue and was creating another blockage. Two more stents were added. Hard to say how much this helped him because he still did not feel well. Prior to the diagnosis of the stent procedure, he kept asking doctors why he felt pain in his upper abdomen area/below his ribs and could not eat anywhere near his normal amount of food, having the always-full-feeling. It hurt him to lay on his side and he complained of dizziness and lethargy. The doctor's aide at the clinic he went to didn't have any answers other than suggesting the heart specialist. The current agenda of the medical industry having its procedures dictated by the insurance industry and Medicare seems to be that it is necessary to treat single issues rather than whole patients. So the Cardiovascular doctor only considered the heart blockage issue. After the stents were installed, he passed Ron along to the next set of doctors. He was sent to a Gastroenterology Lab. A CT scan of his abdomen was ordered.

The Diagnosis

Ron would often walk through the house without his shirt. When he was able to exercise, he liked to walk the neighborhood without a shirt. He was furry. I thought it was funny, our mother was horrified that the neighbors were seeing him so casual. In fact, to paint a full picture for you…..He really liked a pair of teal colored OP corduroy shorts from, I believe, the 1980's. He had large sunglasses, size 12 white sneakers, chicken legs, and a very large upper body with, as I mentioned, an abundant amount of hair. He walked very straight and with authority. Walking the neighborhood, he just seemed like one confident dude. As this was a common look for him, it was easy for me to notice, and it seemed apparent to me that he had a hard lump right up front and center of his gut. So, it didn't come as a surprise that the CT scan showed a suspected Lymphoma. A surgical biopsy was ordered. This required admission to the hospital.

We waited in his hospital room for the official discussion with the doctor. Apparently, it was taking longer because three separate pathologists needed to interpret the results from the biopsy, and all were to be in agreement as to the specifics of the diagnosis. We waited and waited hours past when we were told the doctor would come. Ron, I think, was hoping it was all a mistake. I knew what the diagnosis was going to be; it was just a matter of the kind/stage. Who knows what you really want the demeanor of the doctor to be or what words would be best for them to say? All I know is that I wasn't too thrilled with this doctor. Besides the wait, it just seemed as if he had told this same story so many times that he was no longer phased by it. Anyway, follecular Non-Hodgkin Lymphoma. One mass 12 x 12 x 16cm and several others, the largest being 7.7 x 5.9 cm. We would subsequently refer to them as the *aliens*. It was at least stage 3; they wouldn't know if it was 4 unless they did a bone marrow biopsy. The doctor wrote this in his notes to Ron: "Grade 3a, faster type within the slower growing group. Almost always gets better and stays better for a few to several years. Hard to cure." Treatment was to be BR (Bendamustine and Rituxan) Chemo is hard on the heart and since Ron was compromised in that area, he had to start with this protocol as it was the least damaging chemo cocktail for the heart. Ron was in a complete fog, so I asked the questions. What if he does not do the chemo? So, just ask that question if you want a searing sneer-over-the-glasses-and-down-the-nose-look. The doctor said, "Well, the calcium level would continue to rise until he went into a coma or died." They really don't like it when you question the protocol or even consider that you might not take their suggested treatment. Ron said he needed time to think, and an office visit was scheduled to discuss the treatment further.

While Ron was thinking, I was researching. I read a pretty good book written by an oncologist that explained the history and business behind cancer. Unfortunately, I don't remember the name of it but there is a vast quantity of books and information out there to break it all down.

A great number of books are written for different types of cancer and different treatment angles. It is overwhelming and probably more than you have interest in knowing but I think knowledge is power. In one of the Four Agreement books by the Ruiz family, it says: "Are you controlling the knowledge or is it controlling you?" That's great wisdom to remember.

I gained some knowledge about cancer. First off, it is a very large business to the tune of $158 billion per year (United States Only). Despite that large figure, over 600,000 people die every year from it. An enormous amount of money is spent extending life for a few months. Depending on the type of cancer, a "protocol for treatment" is suggested. There are three types of oncology (cancer) doctors: a medical oncologist (treats with chemo), a surgical oncologist (removal of tumors), and a radiological oncologist (treats with radiation). Treatment can include one or all of those specialties. In the case of Ron's lymphoma, as it was in the lymph system, surgery and radiation were not options. The chemo they suggested was a two-drug cocktail: Bendamustine and Rituximab. Both are used to treat leukemia and lymphoma. Interestingly, Bendamustine was invented in 1963 in East Germany and used there for cancer treatment long before it made its way to the states. It is a nitrogen mustard which was originally used for chemical warfare. Fun….

Someday, society will look back on chemo treatment and scratch their collective heads. A great book if you want some laughs is: ***"Quackery, A Brief History of the Worst Ways To Cure Everything"*** by Lydia Kang, MD

Then if you want a book that should be science fiction but is not: ***"A Crack in Creation"*** by Jennifer Doudna, this is a book written by one of the scientists involved in the origination of CRISPR technology. This is the science of genetically altering RNA. At the time of this writing, they have utilized this technology for the COVID vaccine. I won't even step on that 3rd rail. The reason I mention it is that they are working towards treating some cancers by genetically altering and enhancing a person's immune system. Currently it is very expensive and not widely utilized. Who knows what is possible or where this will go? Time will tell. The power and potential are a little scary.

Alternative Treatments

Ron didn't like the idea of chemo. He thought it was a treatment that killed people. He searched for an alternative. I am all for alternative treatments. If I have a burn, I grab an Aloe Vera plant. I make my own toothpaste with baking soda and Tea Tree Oil. I am a big proponent of considering foods as health aids. Many "old world" cures can be just as effective if not more than any over the counter stuff you can buy. One caveat to natural treatments is that typically, it takes longer to work its magic. If I had the time and a mild case of something I would absolutely treat myself with a natural or alternative approach. Alternative treatments are usually used in place of conventional medicine and include treatments from Homeopath, Naturopaths, or Ayurvedic. There is also what is considered Integrative Therapy. This might mean that along with conventional medical treatment you also practice Tai Chi, use herbs or other supplements, aromatherapy, marijuana, acupuncture, meditation, or chiropractors.

As I was the "researcher" and Ron valued my opinion and looked to me for guidance, I agreed to go with him to a "Wellness Clinic." I don't remember how he knew this doctor, but he had gone to him in the past. He was a Naturopathic physician. His suggestions were to consider Mexican Cancer Clinics (they have less regulations), super high IV doses of Vitamin C (super pricey), and a visit to another doctor that did ultrasound health screenings (would be able to verify or dispute the findings of the hospital's pathology/diagnosis).

From the beginning, I told Ron that I would be there with him every step of the way no matter what he decided, and I was, mostly. He wanted to do the vitamin C infusion treatment. It was very costly and as he didn't have a lot of money, he tried to brainstorm ways to make it happen. I did research the C angle. Again, it might be helpful for some people with mild issues. My feelings that I shared at the time were that if there was any alternative treatment out there that really worked to treat cancer, with the ease of information sharing these days

(Twitter, Facebook, Tickity Tock), what have you, how would this information be kept a secret?

He decided to visit the doctor the naturopath referred him to for a body screening. The outcome was the same, slightly different measurements of the *"aliens"* but same diagnosis. Unfortunately, his determination to treat his cancer naturally was deflated as she agreed that he needed to do chemo.

Going Down Hill

At some point he was tested and found to have "Malignant Ascites." Ascites is the abnormal build-up of fluid in the abdomen. A therapeutic paracentesis was scheduled. (Draining the fluid and in his case with the use of ultrasound)

It had been about six months since Ron had started not feeling well. In retrospect some of this was likely due to the heart valve having some blockage but much of it was the growth of the *"aliens"*. During this time, he had lost about 45 pounds. This was a pretty big change for a guy with the nick name "Moose." In addition to the weight loss, one side effect of the cancer was an increase of calcium in the blood (Hypercalcemia). High levels of calcium really cloud the brain and if high enough can cause a coma. He was sleeping a lot and could barely walk. His first chemo infusions were scheduled for the following week. He was sitting in our mother's wheelchair in the foyer and looked like he could be on a poster for a dying cancer patient. His voice, normally loud and quick, was quiet and slower than someone stoned out of their mind. We made the decision to go the ER. He was admitted.

Starting the Chemo

His calcium was indeed high at over 11 mg/dL (values should be 8.5 - 10.1) so he was given lots of sodium chloride. The decision was made to start his chemo treatment in the hospital rather than wait for the clinic/office visit the following week. He tolerated the chemo treatment (Bendamustin/Rituximab) well and did not seem to have side effects. The suggested treatment would entail infusions two days in a row, once a month, for six months. We were *hopeful*....I drove him to the clinic each time. He could have done these visits on his own, but I didn't want him to be alone. There were people there that were on their own and maybe that was their preference, but I just think it is a crappy thing to go through and not have support. Since he was tolerating the chemo well, he thought he was just going to sail through the whole event. He grew up in the south so he had a way of talking to people, particularly women, that might seem to some as if he was being too friendly, but he really was trying to be light-hearted and bring a little "fun" to a dreary place and process. I think some of the nurses thought he was cute or funny, some probably thought he was obnoxious. After spending so much time with him, I came to realize he was much funnier than I gave him credit for.

Sometimes we were in private rooms but other times we were in an infusion area with several chairs. I would say overall the mood was very somber. I had plenty of time to people watch and was amazed at the vast spectrum. Young, old, thin, heavy, different ethnic backgrounds. There were only a couple that you could pick out of a crowd and identify them as a cancer patient. Just goes to the concept that cancer doesn't discriminate and will attack anyone at any time.

Prior to each chemo visit they run blood tests. Between blood tests, due to the saline IV's he received to keep the calcium level in his blood down, and the chemo treatments, he was feeling a bit like a pin cushion. He chose not to have a PICC line; a peripherally inserted central catheter is a long, thin tube that's inserted through a vein in your arm and passed through to the larger veins near your heart used to give medications. So each time was a new attempt at finding a good vein. Chemo is not friendly to veins, so it got more difficult for the nurses to find a good vein and not poke around. Once he decided to keep the needle in his arm overnight since the next day meant another IV. They started the IV, but it turned out that there was a small blood clot which made his arm hurt badly at the time and for two additional weeks. It had to be removed and a new one inserted in the other arm. He was losing his sense of humor.

Is It Working?

Remember the alternative health screening from before? Ron thought so much of this person and their "technology" that he went back to see how things were going. It was her opinion/diagnosis that the *"aliens"* were shrinking. She suggested that when he finished chemo, he come back and she had a cream that when rubbed on the skin near the "aliens" would draw out the remaining cancer cells. WHAT? If he had skin cancer, I might just buy that, but Lymphoma? He was very happy he was beating this.

His oncologist wanted to find out how things were going. They need to know if the patient should stay on course or change the drug protocol. A CT scan was done. Increased adenopathy (enlargement of lymph nodes). *CRAP!* So, that chemo wasn't working. They wanted another lymph node biopsy to see if the cancer had somehow changed. It had. Now apparently it was aggressive B-Cell Non-Hodgkin Lymphoma. If you like percentages and you want doctors to give them to you, keep in mind they are guessing. Guessing and trying to give you the most positive spin. Placebo has proven to be a big part of healing. If you think you have a high probability of success, that should certainly help you more than being told that you have a poor outlook ahead. At our first cancer meeting, I believe it was 80% for a few to several years of life. (It is not curable and in the best case will come back at some point) Now he dropped to 50%.

A little note on numbers. While they are interesting to know and take into consideration, they are all crap. First off, you are not likely to find the same numbers about anything. Depending on your source, numbers change. How do they know x% of the people experienced something, good or bad? Did everyone let the doctor or hospital know, did that get back to whoever came up with the figure, is it updated? With a previous business I had, I needed to have a survey done for a lawsuit. We hired a professional polling/survey company. The first thing they ask is what do you want the outcome to be? Keep that in mind when you see figures, numbers, percentages; consider the source, and take it with a grain of salt.

The oncologist wanted to know if Ron's cancer was at stage 4, meaning is it in the bone marrow. A bone marrow biopsy was ordered. I went with him for that too. If you don't want to hear your loved one yell out in pain, you may want to sit that one out. Turns out it was only a tiny bit in the marrow, but they still considered it stage 4. The answer was to change the chemo. Due to his heart issues they had to verify the heart health. They did an Echo TransThoracic TTE. Apparently, his heart was just healthy enough for them to give him stronger chemotherapy. Now he would be served an evil cocktail of Cyclophosphamide, Pegfilgrastim, & Rituximab. Yum.

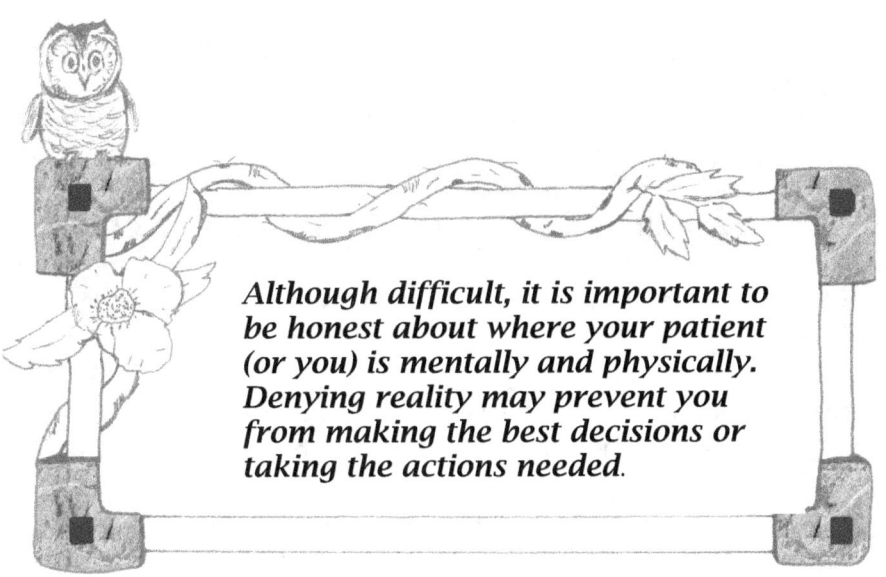

Although difficult, it is important to be honest about where your patient (or you) is mentally and physically. Denying reality may prevent you from making the best decisions or taking the actions needed.

Not So Thankful for Thanksgiving Day

The new Chemo cocktail came with all the side affects you would expect, nausea, lack of appetite, diarrhea, hair loss, generally, a shitty time. BTW, if you have firmly chosen to take the chemo path, don't bother reading the side affects or the warnings because they are unbelievably nasty. They do give you the print outs detailing the drugs so you can read it if you desire. Ron read nothing. I did. One important chemo side effect to monitor was a potential fever. They suggest, if over 100 degrees; go to the ER.

We sat down for the big dinner. Ron didn't look well. He didn't eat which I could absolutely understand. I can't imagine anything tasting like you remembered or even wanting food at all. Food had been a problem for a while. He had no idea what to eat so he just didn't. I kept trying to fix him different meals and initially both mom and I badgered him about the need to eat something, keep your strength up, etc. Apparently, that wasn't correct behavior on my part. Although it is hard to watch them waste away, hounding them about eating increases stress which obviously is not what you want to do.

Not eating wasn't the problem now. He was staring straight ahead, the-nobody's-home-look. When he spoke, it was very quiet, slow and made absolutely no sense at all. I felt his forehead. Fever. So, Thanksgiving night, I spent a few hours at the hospital with him. A battery of tests were ordered, blood, urine, chest Xray, EKG, and brain CT. Diagnosis: Neutropenic fever and Pneumonia. The ER doctor said essentially, he had absolutely no immunities and the absolute worst place for him to be, was the hospital. It was suggested that we leave immediately.

Clearly Ron didn't feel well but I could sense a change while we were there. Gone was his humor to be replaced by a bit of anger. He decided he was done with chemo.

Expectations

From the beginning, I tried to put myself in his shoes. Would I do the chemo? Prior to going through this journey with him, I think I would have said no. After the journey, I know I would say no. As I previously mentioned, I made it clear to him that I would be by his side no matter what he decided, and it was **his** decision. Interestingly, you find out that it is just expected that you are going to do whatever the doctors suggest and, in this case, keep the chemicals flowing. Although Ron had lost his sense of humor by this point, he had a few funny moments. Our mother really didn't understand all that was going on. He was her son and he needed to be healed no matter what it took. Even though the treatments were clearly not working, she said to him, "Maybe you should just go get some more chemo," to which he replied, "You mean like for just shits and giggles?" Maybe you had to be there, but I snort laughed.

People want you to fight, letting life take its course is not the popular view. Other family members, friends, neighbors when told he was not going to continue the treatment, gave a concerned look and said simply; "Oh". Would I want to lose someone close to me "before their time"? No. Expecting anyone to go through chemotherapy or dialysis or any chronic treatments to stay "alive" no matter what state of health it leaves them or at what cost (emotionally and financially) to the family, I think is selfish and lacks empathy. The patient should be able to choose their path and be supported no matter what that path is.

While I was writing this, I happened upon a book at the library, ***"The Unwinding of the Miracle"*** by *Julie Yip-Williams*. It is a memoir of a young women in her 30's that was diagnosed with cancer. In it she thoroughly covers the concept of the struggle not only of the actual treatments themselves but of the back-and-forth mental agony of when to keep fighting and when to let life or death take its course. Is it more courageous to fight to the bitter end or does it take more courage to face your demise head on, accept it, and let the time you have left be **IT?** She experienced and overcame much adversity before the cancer so in her mind giving up wasn't an option. In her case, it was important for her family to know that she did everything imaginable to stay for the most days she could.

I applaud her sheer determination that it took to go through all the different chemotherapy drugs, the radiation, the surgeries, the clinical trials, test after test after test. Yet as I read it, through my paradigm as a caregiver, I couldn't help but think if you added up all the time spent at the hospitals, clinics, recovering, etc. and you deducted that from the total time until death would you be that far off from the time you would have had without the extraordinary measures? Also, as the caregiver, it is heartbreaking to watch your loved one suffer day after day. Again, "hope" is responsible here. First the hope of a cure or remission, then the hope of maybe keeping it at bay for several years, then hope that you can extend your life for a year, months, weeks. We all hope for outcomes that "win" the game. Sometimes the underdog pulls out a miracle and sometimes a sure thing goes in the toilet. She also describes the utter mental devastation and collapse every time the new treatment failed, or the test showed increased cancer. It is as if hope sends you up in a hot air balloon and reality shuts off the wind and you plummet to the ground. I am aware that when dealing with people and emotions it seems cold to suggest that hope be put to the side for a moment while reality is considered, but I think it is a valid process even if you ultimately decide to go all the way down hope's road.

Ron circled back to visit the alternative health screening doctor; it seems she had to admit that although last time the "aliens" were shrinking and things were great, now things were bad, and it was also her opinion/diagnosis that he should continue the chemo. He didn't want to hear that and for awhile he believed that he might just be able to positive attitude his way out of this.

Hope makes you choose certain paths in life. Initially, we all had hoped that he would get beyond this, but things had changed. One day we were sitting together, and he was clearly having a discouraging day. I said, "I am sorry. I don't know what to say." He replied, "There are no words". The hope was gone. Now all that was ahead was decline.

The Decline

Maybe it's because I am just a pessimist much of the time, but from the beginning I didn't have a good feeling about Ron winning this one. After the original diagnosis and subsequent reading about Lymphoma, I really thought he would die within a short period of time. I didn't have any time frame in mind but none the less the monkeys in my brain began to process that. How bad will he get, how long will he be sick, what will I do after, how will I take care of mom, how will mom get through this, etc. etc. So, when the first round of chemo initially looked as if the tumors (aliens) were shrinking, I had to back track. The pessimist was wrong again (I often went to negative land and almost always didn't need to). He was going to get through this. Ok, so now I will process that. I no longer need to think about all that stuff flowing through my head about him not being in our lives. I could start thinking about a future life that included Ron. The roller coaster went down then it was headed back up.

Coasters don't stay at the top. Ron continued to lose weight; he became confused about simple things. Using his computer and phone became at first difficult then impossible. His confusion was my clarity that he was on his way out. The mental/emotional roller coaster is a brutal ride. There is nothing I could write or that you could read that will prepare you for the heartbreak of watching someone you care about breakdown mentally and physically.

When it was clear that Ron wasn't going to do more chemo, I didn't know what to expect but I knew I would need help. I talked to him about Hospice. He didn't want it. I tried to explain that it wasn't just for him but for me. He finally agreed that I could call a Home Health/Hospice company. A nurse came out and chatted with us. Ron's demeanor was strange. He had a weird smirk on his face and wouldn't really answer the questions. Later, I found out that apparently, he didn't think she was really a nurse, didn't like her, yada yada. Did I mention confusion?? Anyway, I agreed to call a different firm but made it clear I wouldn't continue to call every company in the valley. We signed up with the next firm.

Ron had a daughter and granddaughter. They lived about 3 hours away visiting infrequently, some holidays or birthdays. They had not been apart of his journey. I made it very clear to his daughter that if she wanted any meaningful conversation with her father that she needed to visit him immediately. If you find yourself in a similar situation with your loved one mentally declining, trust that you will know "when" they hit that wall or point of no return. Do your best to make sure anyone that matters is informed so that they get the chance to "say goodbye" or if not good with finality, at least a-you-are-cared-for-hug.

A couple of years prior we had moved our mother down to the main floor (more on that later) and Ron's room was at the top of the stairs. He did not have enough energy to come down the stairs and definitely not to get back up. We tried a hospital bed on the main floor, but he would not sleep on it. So, he was "trapped" upstairs. Meanwhile our mother, knowing her son was dying, was "trapped" on the main floor. Despite her inability to walk without a walker and her primary transport a wheelchair, I believe it was four occasions that she climbed the fourteen stairs to sit with her son. You want to talk about a heart wrenching moment. Well-beyond-Hallmark.

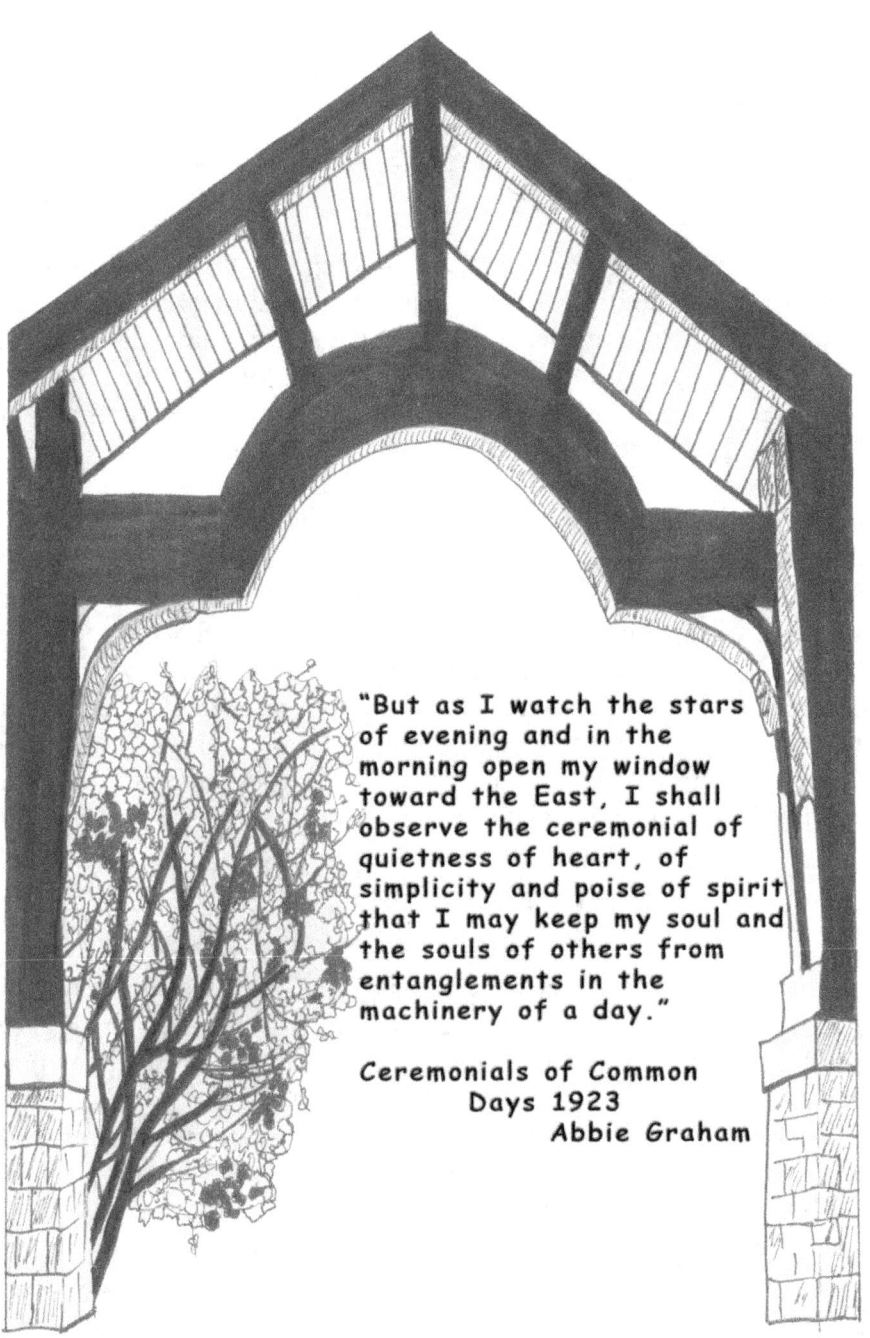

"But as I watch the stars of evening and in the morning open my window toward the East, I shall observe the ceremonial of quietness of heart, of simplicity and poise of spirit that I may keep my soul and the souls of others from entanglements in the machinery of a day."

Ceremonials of Common Days 1923
Abbie Graham

Chapter Five

Hospice

Most people think of hospice as an organization that gets involved at the very end. Of course, many people that utilize the service are in the final stages. It is considered palliative care to help with care and comfort for those with typically less than six months to live. It can be reviewed and continued longer than six months if necessary, and you can cancel their service anytime you want.

Choosing hospice care means that you have chosen not to continue life saving measures. (Note that hospice care received in the hospital setting is a different situation) They do not typically give IV's and some medications may be up to you to continue purchasing separately. If your person gets pneumonia or has a heart attack, by having hospice you are agreeing that you are not calling 911 or going to the ER. You can certainly choose to do that, but it will then cancel the hospice service. It is best to make your mind up on this topic before calling them in. (More on hospice later)

Advanced Directives

In general, advanced directives (living will) are legal papers stating what level of life saving measures you want. Neither of my patients would even answer the questions let alone have the official paper notarized. I got, "I don't care, you decide." Arhgggg
It shouldn't be up to anyone but you if you want to be on a respirator with limited brain activity or if you are ok with a feeding tube rammed up your nose. If you can get these documents filled out early on, you should. Here is a website that may be helpful with FAQ's www.intermountainhealthcare.org/health-information/advance-directive/

Durable Power of Attorney for Health Care (sometimes known as the medical power of attorney). This document would make you the agent and give you the power to make health decisions if there is not a living will. This power of attorney doesn't have anything to do with financial matters. If you need to have access and control to financials, secure a (POA). A power of attorney (POA) or letter of attorney is a written authorization to represent or act on another's behalf in private affairs, business, or some other legal matter. The person authorizing the other to act is the principal, grantor, or donor (of the power). Once the person dies the POA is no longer valid.

POLST (Physician Orders for Life-Sustaining measures)
Hospice will require this document. If for some reason emergency medical is called, they need to know what level of care they can administer and can not use the advanced directive for that.

NOTE: It is important to consider that in all areas of financial and legalities, every state can have different laws/rules and you should consult your specific state information.

Hospice Continued...
When and why to get them involved? Unfortunately, death doesn't always happen quick and painlessly or neat and tidy. In my brother Don's case, it did. He fell over and that was it. The paramedics toted him away to the hospital and then the funeral home picked him up from the hospital. Logistically, simple. Basically, he died at home and since he wasn't being treated currently for any medical issues, they did an autopsy to rule out any foul play. Hospice skips that necessity.

If end of life care were as easy as feeding and propping up pillows for your loved one, you could handle it by yourself. Unfortunately, simple things like walking, showering, or visiting the toilet can get very challenging. If you have several people involved in caretaking, then you might not need hospice until the very end if at all. The three main things they are good for are providing medications, primarily morphine, pronouncing the person officially deceased, and bringing in durable medical equipment if needed. (beds, oxygen, chairs, etc.)

In addition to morphine there are other medications that may be required to assist with agitation, sleep, nausea, lung congestion, etc. The nurse will assess the patient as well as consult with you to make the patient more comfortable and or easier for you to handle. Since the patient is unlikely to be able to go to doctor's appointments, this is a way to get medications without leaving the home. I will discuss medications later.

I wanted them to tell me what to expect. They wouldn't and couldn't. Too many variables. Anything can happen. The hospice packet included information on weeks, days, hours, before death. It was somewhat helpful to read, but you really just have to ride the daily wave.

Depending on your particular situation, hospice might be very helpful and perhaps you won't have other options, but they also might be very disappointing. Like any business, some are better than others. And they are a business…..

Despite any negative experiences I might have had with hospice, I do need to say that the nurses that have chosen hospice care are special people. I said to one, "It must be difficult to be a hospice nurse given that all of your patients eventually die". To which she replied, "A specialty such as obstetrics has the opportunity to bring people into the world and I get the opportunity to help them out of the world." Such a great attitude.

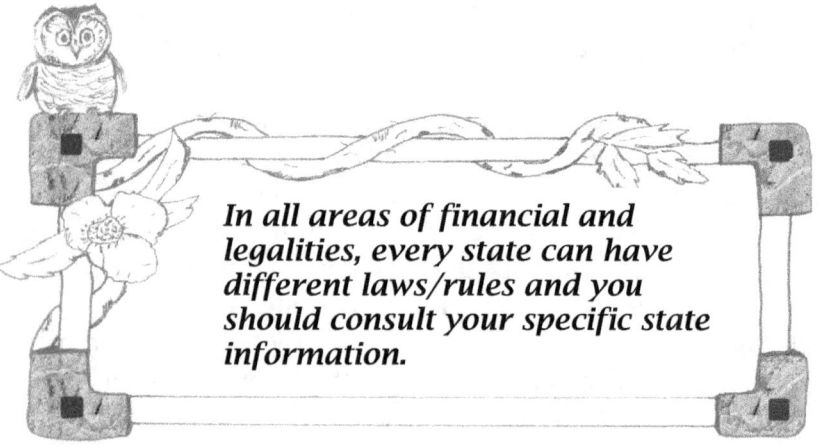

In all areas of financial and legalities, every state can have different laws/rules and you should consult your specific state information.

In Hospital Hospice

Years ago, there were centers dedicated to hospice care. Now, when people talk about hospice it is usually home assistance. Recently, I was aware of two separate situations where hospice within the hospital was utilized. In the first case, my friend's husband had been admitted to the hospital with an infection. The infection was out of control, and he exhibited a scary level of agitation. When it became apparent that taking him home was not an option, the hospital suggested their hospice program. The same care as home hospice would be given for a short-term period of 3 to 5 days. Keep the patient as comfortable as possible but not continue life saving measures. He was given a large room where family and friends could stay with him or just say their goodbyes. The second case was my partner's father who at the time was 86 and had been sleeping for most of every day. He was admitted to the hospital because he had fallen and wasn't very coherent. After numerous tests, the emergency room doctor said that nothing was wrong or more precisely, nothing was treatable so they would be unable to keep him. During the few hours of testing, he had become unresponsive. It was still their suggestion to either send him home or to a long-term care facility. Home was not an option, and it didn't seem like he was going to be long term. A social worker was brought in to evaluate him which ultimately resulted in hospice being called in to take over his care while remaining at the hospital. He passed away the second day.

Not all hospitals have this program but they all should. According to the hospice nurse, it is evaluated case by case, but the patient does need to have out of control anxiety or pain. In his case, the unresponsiveness was also a reason they agreed to bring in hospice. In both examples, taking the patient home was just not a possibility, a rehab center is only good if the person is able to rally and continue improving and long-term care is very expensive and in both of these cases, not necessary.
If you feel like you are in a similar situation, ask to speak to a social worker to help you with the solution that is best for you.

Back to Ron

I tried to make his room as pleasant as possible for him. I hung some of his pictures we got from his storage unit, played music from his MP3, aroma therapy diffuser, extra pillows, etc. Brought him something for breakfast, lunch, and dinner. Most was left uneaten. One thing he would usually eat was my home bottled fruit. He liked the peaches. Refilled his ice water, administered his morphine. Although I was the primary on the care, I wasn't alone. We had another brother who stopped by on a regular basis to check on Ron and to help with our mother (more on that later). The hospice service provides for a CNA to come in once or twice a week. They can assist with showering. To be fair, that is likely not a job that people are clamoring to get. Ron also wanted a male so that further limited the options. The CNA didn't speak English very well so that made it a bit challenging. Ron made it to the shower twice with the CNA and then there was one sponge bath. This wouldn't have been a long-term viable option. Maybe a different person would have made a difference??

At this stage, I was going home at night. I wondered when it would get to a point where he could not be left alone. I would imagine everyone will encounter a situation or event that answers that question. I had one.

Round the Clock Care

Every morning when I opened the door, I wondered what would be waiting for me on the other side. Would he be dead? What state would my mother be in? This morning upon entering, my mother was very upset and said Ron had been yelling for hours. Her time clock was all screwed up by this point, so I didn't have any way of knowing how long he had been yelling but he was indeed yelling. I flew up the stairs and tried the door. There was something in the way preventing it from opening all the way. Ron used to own an old Greyhound scenic cruiser bus. It was a treasure for him. Years prior he was forced to sell it. He had a very large-framed poster of a Scenic Cruiser and I had added that to his room. It was on the wall right as you entered. Well, that was where it was the night before, now it was on the floor, partially on top of him. Fortunately, the glass had not broken. None the less, although there were other heartbreaking moments over the previous weeks, this one was off the scale……..he was on the floor, naked, yelling that he was trapped. The framed bus picture was partially on top of him. Keep in mind that my big brother "Moose" now weighed less than me and frankly looked like a Holocaust victim. I picked him up from the floor, got him back to bed and eventually in a calm state. It is hard to keep your sense of humor when you are caring for someone. I tried to keep mine during and after. Whenever I discuss with someone the topic of my longevity on the planet, I say the same tag line. After I got Ron situated, I thought to myself, "Well, you can always get hit by a bus." A little levity after an emotional typhoon. And there was the answer to my question: I would be staying the night.

The Call of Nature

If you go through an ending that isn't quick, your person and their need to pee is going to be an issue. I don't know if it is that the body plays tricks, or they forget they just went or just that nothing is working right, but chances are they are not drinking enough to need to pee as often as they think they do. Ron wouldn't or couldn't use the bedside potty or the plastic urinal. That meant he had to get up and walk to the bathroom and with his little toothpick legs and lack of energy, made a simple trip to the toilet a difficult event. During the day things seem to go a bit smoother; night was a different story. I was in the next room so I could hear him when he stirred. Consequently, I didn't get much sleep. I dozed off briefly when I heard him yell. The first time, I bounced out of bed to run to his aid. Not a great idea. I am in my 50's in pretty decent shape, but I thought I might just have a heart attack. The room swirled and I had to grab the wall for a few seconds. For subsequent events, I sat for a few before bounding down the hall. Anyway, he was yelling, "Son of a bitch; I got to pee." As he yelled, he was trying to get up by rocking back and forth, head on pillow, feet in air, then slam the feet down, head off of pillow. He just didn't have the strength to get to a standing position which I guess was good because he would have just landed on the floor. It would have been so much easier if he could have used the bedside options but…

Help from Others

Maybe it's just me. Since I had been "in-charge" of Ron, I apparently became possessive of my patient. There were people I could have asked to assist me, but since I was already in the house taking care of our mother; what's another patient? Towards the end, since I knew time was limited, I wanted to be there and spend the time. But I also still had my own home life to manage (more on that later). This is one of my suggestions under the heading of "things I would do differently." Although I may have been taking great care of Ron, others can provide care as well. It also gives them time to "be" with the person.

Now he had gotten to the point of not being able to get up. This meant diapers. Life's cruel little circle back to the beginning. Only now you are aware of the total dependance on other humans and the humiliation of needing this service. We had the hospice nurse come in and give us the tutorial on changing an adult's diaper, but I have to say, it is not an easy process. Over time, one could get the hang of it, but it is a challenge. Fortunately, or unfortunately depending on how you look at it, we didn't have to struggle with it for very long.

Again, you can read the information they give you on the last days, but my advice is to just be patient and tackle each day with whatever it brings. In Ron's case it was apparent that it would be any time now.

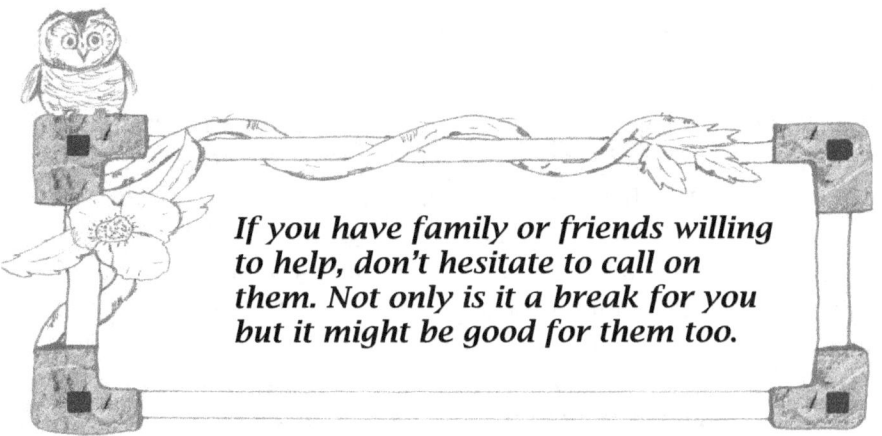

If you have family or friends willing to help, don't hesitate to call on them. Not only is it a break for you but it might be good for them too.

The Road Home

It was evening. The whole family was crammed into his bedroom. He hadn't really communicated in a couple of days. Earlier in the day the nurse had said his vitals were still pretty good. Now breathing was shallow and sporadic. They talk about "The Death Rattle," a sound often produced by someone who is near death when fluids such as saliva and bronchial secretions accumulate in the throat and upper chest. He didn't really do much of this, mostly decreased breathing until it was maybe a couple of breaths per minute.

We thought he was gone. Then suddenly his eyes opened, and he gasped for breath. It was like a scary movie. I don't think anyone screamed but it was a little creepy. There is a funny line in the movie, "Princess Bride," when Billy Crystal says, "no he is only mostly dead." So that was Ron for a minute, then he was really dead. A friend of mine's husband had the doctor pronounce him. His daughter went over and put her hand on his chest, and he started breathing again and for several more hours. Some people just fight leaving on that final journey. Whatever you feel that is.

We called the hospice company, and the nurse came out. The nurse did the official "pronouncement" and cleaned up the body and called the funeral home. Since it was late night, they scheduled a morning pickup.

Funerals, Cemeteries, Cremations

When Don died, we were at a loss of what to do. As I mentioned, I had been nominated family get-it-done person, so I just crossed one little bridge at a time. When you are younger, you don't think about any of this stuff (at least not everyone does). We didn't. I knew Don was an atheist. He never had a specific discussion about his "ending" with anyone, and it probably wouldn't have mattered because he did not have a living will and his mother wanted him to have a funeral and to be buried. Another reason why you might like to get a "Living Will." The atheist had a really nice Mormon service/funeral.

I had a referral of a funeral home that was reasonably priced, and Ron and I picked out a fairly conservatively priced casket for Don. Because we now had breached the dreaded subject, I was able to get both Ron and our mother to agree that they both wanted funerals and to be buried so I purchased three plots together in a small quaint local cemetery.

I learned that if you are going to go with cremation, you can likely get that done for under $1,500. Even though it is just going in the fire, the body still must be in a box, so depending on what you select, that can make a difference in price. Of course, the "urn" or similar ash container choice will make a difference.

For burials, in addition to the coffin and plot of land, you also need to purchase a cement vault for the casket to live in and there is the fee by the cemetery for the actual burial. As conservative as we were it was still around $9,000. Add another $800+ for the headstone.

Here is what frustrates me about funerals, in addition to the financial and emotional toll and clown makeup on the dead person. Why do people show up that you haven't seen in years? If they cared about the person, why have they never called? Did they really even know the deceased? They certainly weren't there for difficult times. If they were sent a note in advance that the person was dying, would they have called or stopped by then? Strange customs we have.

I have heard about people doing a pre-funeral. They know the end is near and before it gets to the ugly stage, they throw their last party. Great idea. Rather than everyone getting together telling stories about the dead person and sending flowers that will be dead soon as well, reminisce with the dying person, have some laughs, some hugs, good music, food, alcohol, etc. You get a chance to say what you need to say, no should-a, could-a, would-a's. They get a chance to spend some time with the people in their life that really mattered (otherwise they wouldn't have been invited). If I know in advance and I have friends still alive at that point, I am going with the pre-funeral party plan.

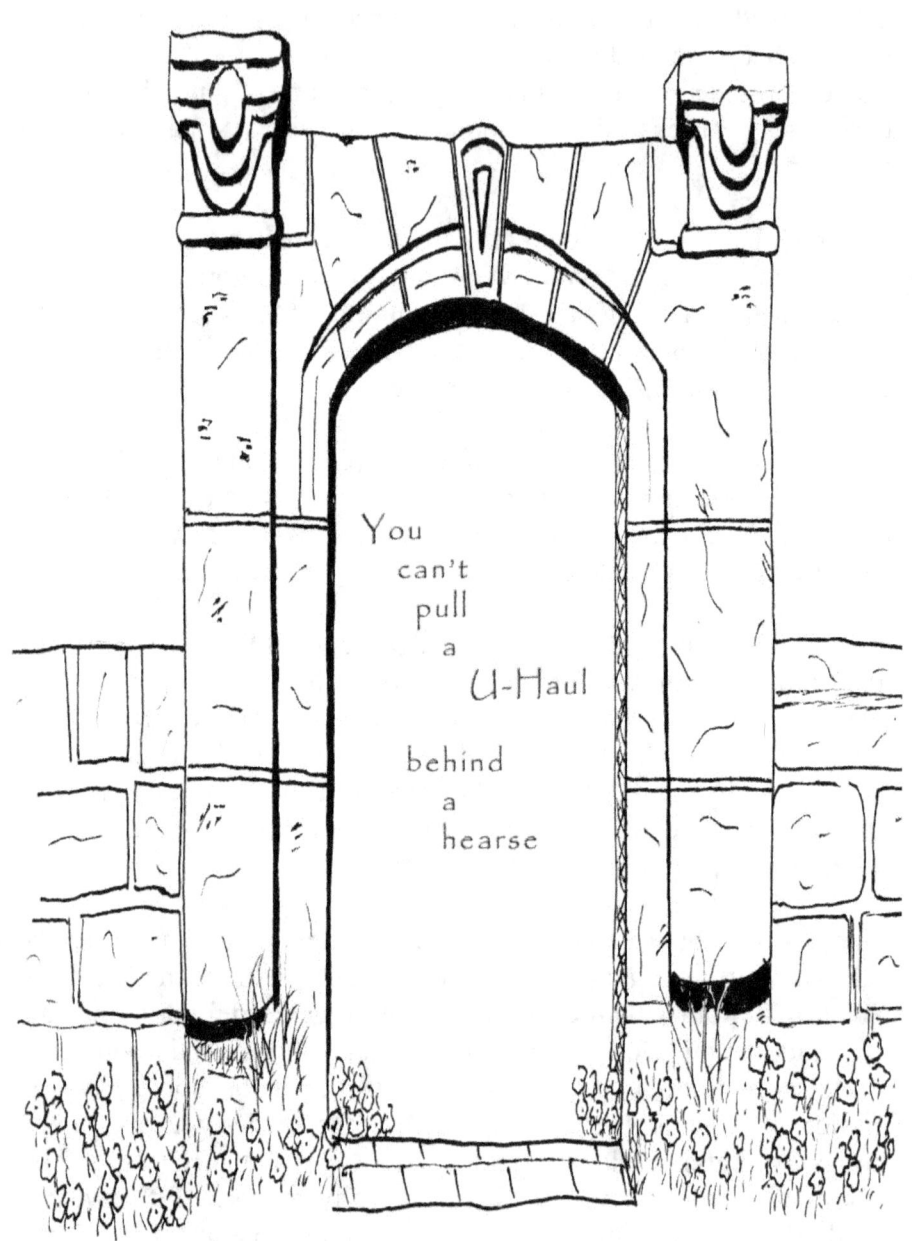

The Stuff

It is interesting that we spend our whole life hunting, gathering, and storing stuff. Collectibles, clothes, cars, practical things, useless things, lots of things and we spend lots of money and stress to get those things. In the end, none of it matters. Unless your relatives want to throw down over the things, then maybe it matters. Some Native American tribes bury the prized possessions with the person then burn the rest. That's interesting. No reason to acquire huge quantities of stuff and nothing for anyone to bicker about. Most of us are collectors.

When Don died, it took Ron and me months to go through everything. He was the step beyond collecting. Hoarding. He had a path to his bed but other than that, the floor was filled with "stuff," Papers, receipts, electronics (mostly dead), books, magazines, clothes, (some brand new with tags), gifts he received (unused and unopened), trash, etc. Dusting hadn't happened in at least twenty years, and he smoked. Needless to say, a good share went in the trash or recycle, several trips to second hand, a few things to relatives, and a very few things were sold. I wondered what made him live like that. We had all seen his room but not until we actually went through it did I find myself so disturbed by it. If you are interested in the topic, there is a great book: ***"Stuff, Compulsive Hoarding and the Meaning of Things" by Randy Fost and Gail Steketee.*** This book has great history and insights, but I still would have to guess what started him on that path.

Ron had lots of stuff, much of which had been living at a large storage unit for the previous three years. He had intended to get his own place, but it just never happened. A couple of weeks before he died, he insisted I drive him to the storage unit. He looked at his "stuff" and viewed it as the culmination of his life and didn't feel that he had amounted to anything. He had tears in his eyes, it was very emotional, and it saddened me that he felt that his life had anything to do with stuff that he would leave behind.

As I mentioned earlier, he had a daughter, and I just assumed she would inherit everything and deal with it. Nope. After repeated attempts at getting her to do so, I realized I would be dealing with everything. I did have the presence of mind to get him to sign the titles to his two cars before he died which made it easy for me to sell those. One thing I did not do prior to his cognitive decline was get his passwords and account information. Towards the end, he could not remember them, and he did not have any of it written down.

I methodically went through everything. Because I had his funeral to pay for, I was hoping to generate some cash. I utilized eBay for quite a bit of my research. I looked up the item to see how much it sold for. Note that what things are listed for isn't the true figure you need. There is a box you can check on the left-hand side of the screen for listing only the items actually sold. Sometimes there is a huge difference.

My method was to first take anything I wanted to keep and have my other brother do the same. Then I would determine if it would have enough value to bother posting on eBay given the fees, shipping, etc. I also posted some things that were too large to ship on a local internet based classified site. Nieces also had a chance to go through items. Here's what I learned about selling things. *Shit ain't worth shit.* I am sure everyone has seen at least one episode of Antique Road Show. There is always a super ugly vase that goes for thousands or a toy worth hundreds. Good luck to you if you find a needle in the haystack in your loved one's stuff and then good luck to you to find someone willing to shell out hundreds or thousands for it.

I wasn't doing it full time as I was taking care of my mother, but it took me almost a year to process everything. In the aggregate, I was able to generate enough for the funeral and a little extra to help me with my expenses since I had become a full-time care giver without a salary. More on "stuff" later.

Down to One Patient

Prior to Ron becoming ill, he had been a great help to me in taking care of our mother. Since he lived in her house, he was there evenings and weekends, so I didn't have to worry about her during those times. I did anyway of course. This brings up one of my top "if I had to do it over" words of wisdom to share. Take advantage of those willing or able to help. I don't mean that in a negative sense. Taking care of someone becomes very consuming of your time and emotions. Early on is your time to take breaks, vacations, or just time away from the environment. Later it may be either physically or mentally difficult for you to take any time for yourself. Don't feel guilty even if your "patient" tries to gift you with a matching set of guilt bags on your way out. They will get over it and even if the "sub" doesn't do things how or as wonderful as you would, it is unlikely that anyone will perish during the time you are gone.

I was already several years into the caregiving before I realized I missed the boat on taking breaks, vacations, etc. I think it sneaks up on you. Again, with hindsight it all becomes much clearer. As I mentioned earlier, my mother had her own business and had built a building next to her house to accommodate it. Despite my being adamant about not wanting to do this business, I found myself doing it anyway. That's another irrelevant story. Over the years I had done some paperwork for her, but I found myself doing most of the financial work for her business. She had always said she thought she would die at her desk. Of course, she meant she would never retire. It was obvious, though, that she did not want to do this work any longer and I couldn't blame her. So, she wasn't staying in the office as long, then gradually not at all. No concerns there. The concern started with repeated mistakes in her check register, leaving bills in a folder, not paying them, and incurring late fees.

Financial Concerns

I already had a Power of Attorney for my mom as I had to pay her bills while she was out of the country years before for an extended time. Now this topic made me uneasy. I had taken over the business, organically. It wasn't orchestrated or even talked about. I didn't want my mother to feel like I was taking away her independence or have any suspicions that I might "take the money and run." Many seniors have good cause to be suspect.

My name was added to her checking accounts so that I could pay bills or access money if needed. I did not add my name to credit cards, and I would suggest that you not do that either or you will be on the hook for the bill when they die. The mortgage was in her name only, and adding my name would have required rewriting the loan and we did not want to do that. If you want to avoid probate, you may want to consider adding your name to the mortgage. Even if you are the executor of a will leaving the house to you, it does not prevent the need for probate if the house is in the deceased's name only. You might also consider, assuming all parties agree to it, quitclaim the property to a trustworthy heir. If the property has a mortgage, you may need to check on the terms. Also, if you are devesting the property to qualify for Medicaid, you must do that five years prior to applying for any Medicaid benefits.

Another financial topic that I dreaded discussing was that we were going to have a running-out-of-money problem. The business wasn't doing that great; it seemed as if I wasn't making a lot more than what it cost to run. When I added that up and combined the stress of doing the job and the stress of taking care of my mother, I needed to be done with it. My ideas for money options were few. We still had some of Don's life insurance money at the time, Ron was still with us, but he just had his social security so the only option I could see was considering a reverse mortgage.

Reverse Mortgages

There is a lot of negative press out there about Reverse Mortgages and I can see why. If the homeowner lives a long time you will eat up all the equity. The house is first appraised and based on that figure, they determine how much money you can get out of it. There are fees involved. Every month the money you owe will increase as interest accrues. You are allowed to take a percentage of the equity at the time of the loan but will need to wait for one year to take out additional money. You can also set it up for a monthly payment or draw rather than taking lump sums. The house is still the owner's property, and all upkeep and expenses will still need to be paid.

A couple of negatives to consider: if the person lives for a long time there will be no equity, although the heirs will not owe money if the balance is greater than the value. They will tell you that you have up to one year after the homeowner leaves the property (either to a care facility or death) to sell the property and pay back the loan. This isn't quite as straight forward as it sounds. You have to show that you are actively selling the home within the first 90 days. If you can, then they can issue another 90 days extension and repeat up to the year. (More on this later)

In our case, we did not have a choice financially. You will want to investigate your options thoroughly before going with this option.

https://www.hud.gov/program_offices/housing/sfh/hcc/reverse_mortgages1

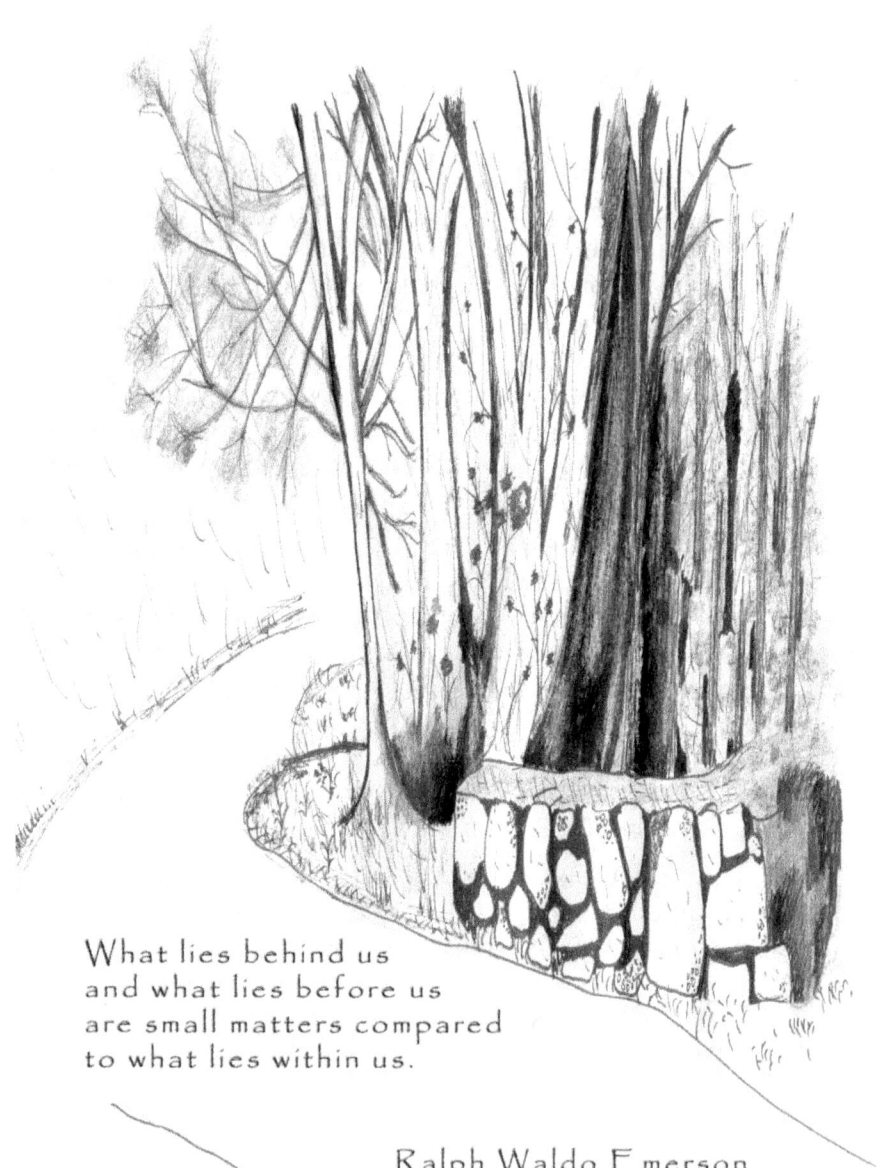

What lies behind us
and what lies before us
are small matters compared
to what lies within us.

Ralph Waldo Emerson

Chapter Six

Back To The Mom

There was a lot of medical "stuff" that my mother had been enduring for several years, so I was not surprised that her mental capacity was affected. Perhaps it was just aging, who knows.

It had been seventeen years of struggling with her balance and feeling of constant motion. Everything imaginable was done to get at the root cause. Multiple brain MRI's, balance clinic, ear testing, spinal tap, blood tests, EMG (Electromyography: measures muscle response or electrical activity in response to a nerves stimulation of the muscle), optical tests, EKG (Electrocardiogram: a test that measures the electrical activity of the heartbeat. What they came up with was "accelerated microvascular disease." Essentially teeny tiny little strokes that can damage the brain. Secondary to that was Leukoaraiosis (increased white matter in the brain). The strange thing was they also said that the damage was not in the area of the brain that handles balance. At least they tried to come up with answers. Years prior, my grandmother complained of feeling "woosey," She was told, "Old people get dizzy." Perhaps she had the same issue as my mother. We will never know. And I hope to hell I won't be experiencing it. I get car, plane, bus, boat sick, I haven't ridden on amusement rides that go in circles in years, and virtual motion/video games make my head spin. If I had to go through every day of my life feeling like that, I would have to find a way out. Frankly, I don't know how my mother did it.

So, the imbalance issue was huge, but it was certainly not all that her body was subject to. In the 90's she had both hips replaced. The surgeon was excellent, all went well, and she was a trooper with rehab. She traveled extensively, walked, swam, was always active. In the last four years of her life, she had a very difficult time getting up from a chair. The doctors couldn't see any reason for it. She had stopped her normal exercising as the balance issue and failing eyesight made it difficult. I wonder if having artificial hips or knees require you to be more vigilant about maintaining leg strength. I don't know, but based on how difficult it became for my mother, I practice getting out of a chair and off the floor without using my hands and I would advise everyone to do the same.

Procedures that were less invasive and seemingly without repercussions include several injections of hylan G-F 20 for the knee (one of the most common types of joint lubricant injections used for the treatment of knee arthritis). There was a one-time Synvisc brand injection off-label for a shoulder, cataract surgery, LRTI (thumb surgery, total waste of time and money), broken ankle, a tummy tuck (while there may not have been any obvious repercussions from this, it was also a waste of time and money and in no way worth the risk of the surgery. While I know that it was ultimately my mother's decision, I question the ethics of the surgeon agreeing to the surgery for a woman in her mid-70's.)

Shoulder Replacement and a Few Bumps In the Road

In 2008, my mother had her right shoulder replaced. The surgery went very well, and I remember her being particularly happy about the pain pump she had in the hospital. I am sure there are a lot of people who would like one of those for home use. Even after they took that away, she didn't have much pain. Due to her balance issue, it was suggested she go to a care center to rehab rather than going straight home. Here's where things went south.

The care center was less than two blocks away from her home and our office, so I walked there everyday sometimes twice. That is the only thing good I have to say about it. She complained that she was constipated. Who doesn't hate when that happens? Rather than being patient for the after-surgery pain meds to dissipate and her system to return to normal, she continued to complain to the staff. So, they gave her Milk of Magnesia (MOM). I don't have any idea how much, but she called me close to midnight saying she was in extreme pain. Apparently, they were not equipped to handle the situation, so she was transported in an ambulance back to the hospital. No need for extra graphics but apparently on the way, there was a shit-storm. We spent several hours in an ER evaluation room where shit continued to rain down. It wasn't pretty. I don't know if it is accurate or not, but the nurse in the ER said she shouldn't have been given the MOM. Clearly it didn't work out well. They had to make sure there were no medical issues, so they did a scan, the type of which I don't remember. Eventually, a couple of doctors came in to alarm us unnecessarily. They saw "something" they didn't like on the scan that might need emergency surgery. X$#@*&. I called Ron to update him on Mom's status, and he came up to the hospital to sit and stress with me. After another hour or so of more waiting, the consensus was that it wasn't anything significant after all, maybe just a little scar tissue. Perhaps they could have come to that consensus prior to mentioning the need for emergency surgery. Anyway, that issue put to bed, the tests showed she had c-diff so she was admitted to the hospital for IV antibiotics. (Also known as *Clostridioides difficile* or *C. difficile*) it is a germ (bacterium) that causes severe diarrhea and colitis (an inflammation of the colon). An interesting factoid that I didn't know at the time: according to the CDC, one in 11 people over age 65 diagnosed with a healthcare-associated *C. diff* infection die within one month. Kind of glad I didn't research that bit of trivia during the event. And if all that wasn't enough fun, she also acquired a case of Shingles. At some point Ron was discussing Mom's Shingles (don't remember why, slow news day perhaps), but he couldn't remember what they were called so he called them Skittles. Not to belittle the potential life-altering affliction but we continued to refer to them as Skittles. In no way as enjoyable as the tasty little fruit candies.

From the Head to the Heart

My mother was fairly progressive and knowledgeable about the medical industry having worked with medical companies during her many years as a recruiter/headhunter. Her neurosurgeon, I would have to say, was the most personable and seemingly caring doctor that I encountered throughout all of her and Ron's healthcare journeys. He was also very progressive and did a lot of research regarding neuro issues. My mother was hopeful that perhaps treatment with stem cells would be available to her for treatment of the microvascular disease or the Leukoaraiosis. Unfortunately, as he would explain, although stem cell therapy showed promise in certain applications, neuro wasn't one of them. She asked about a clinical trial. There was not one that he was aware of. Clinical Trials are sort of the hail Mary. You agree to be a lab rat for a medical or pharmaceutical company to try new drugs or procedures that "might" help you live longer. With pharmaceuticals they are usually "blind" studies meaning you might get the drug or you might get a placebo. They are a last-ditch effort and are very expensive for the companies, so they are usually only conducted at major hospitals in certain areas of the country.

Around 2014 the neurosurgeon was out of ideas at least neurologically speaking. He detected an abnormal heart rhythm, so he suggested a heart monitor for a week. These are annoying little boxes with leads attached to you that you wear for a week. They record the heart beats and any stops and starts are red flagged. So called, "episodes." The monitor registered some of these episodes, so the neuro passed the baton to the cardio.

Atrial Fibrillation (A-FIB)

She was referred to a cardiac doctor specializing in electrophysiology (studies the electrical properties of biological cells and tissues). According to his expert opinion, the heart monitor showed that she had a few "episodes" and therefore she was diagnosed with A-Fib (irregular heartbeat). The neurologist had already prepared me for this likely outcome, and he also mentioned the drugs they typically prescribed to treat it. They prescribe anticoagulants, not to be confused with blood thinners. The theory is that with A-Fib, the heart has "episodes" where it stalls then starts back up. There is a potential that if you had a small clot of blood when it started back up, it would "throw" the clot and potentially cause a stroke. The general view is that if you have A-Fib you are at a greater risk for stroke. It is difficult to find a consensus on how great your risk is, and it obviously depends on your overall health and medical history. Anyway....I had already researched the drug issue before the doctor's appointment. So, I wasn't surprised when he suggested the "new" drug. (I.E. more expensive and not as much documentation on side effects). I am not sure who I didn't like more, Ron's oncologist or this guy. Either way, they were not interested in anyone questioning their diagnosis or treatment. My mother had already started being too quiet or not giving the correct answers during doctor's visits, so I took it upon myself to be the devil's advocate. I said she already took aspirin. "Not working," he said. One of the drugs he prescribed was Diltiazem which is a calcium channel blocker. Although all drugs have side effects, this one I wasn't as concern about. The new anti-coagulant drug he wanted her to have was Eliquis (Apixaban). The research I had done explained that this drug did not have an "antidote," meaning if there was an accident leading to blood loss, it could be a real problem. One of the side effects is dizziness (already a problem) and another potential, wait for it......a stroke. To be clear, I didn't want her to take any anti-coagulant, but this is what they prescribe, and they make the patient scared not to take it. I said she should take the "old" drug which is Warfarin. He wasn't happy but he wrote the prescription. Again, I wasn't happy about this drug either. Warfarin has been around a long time and happens to have originally been used as rat poison. Was it the lesser of two evils, who knows? If the patient has a history of falling, you might want to really think this one over. Fortunately, my mother did not fall often and amazingly enough she never got the thin skin that happens after long term use. A friend of mine's husband developed extremely thin skin and fell A LOT. Not always, but many times it meant a trip to the ER to get the blood to stop. The slightest scratch from the dog or a bump into something resulted in a major open wound. I don't remember how long my mother took the Warfarin but it proved to be a pain in the ass. It requires testing of the person's INR (international normalized ratio) or basically, clotting factor. The INR can be influenced by foods that are eaten so it is extremely difficult to maintain the ideal rate. The dose had to constantly be changed. She didn't want to keep doing the testing, so Eliquis happened anyway.

Drugs: Cost Assistance and Considerations

Warfarin was cheap, Eliquis was not. Depending on your insurance, the co-pays can really add up for the newer pricier drugs. It is not always possible, but you may want to reach out to the manufacturer of the drug and see what they offer. After contacting Bristol Myers Squibb, the manufacturer of Eliquis, we were able to get the drug at a reduced rate. Later, when we changed Medicare supplemental companies, the co-pay was basically the same amount, so it made it unnecessary to go through BMS. If you have Medicare and are enrolled in a Part D plan, you can request extra help for co-pays. If you or your patient take a lot of medication the costs add up quick. Take a look at the Medicare site:
https://www.ssa.gov/benefits/medicare/prescriptionhelp.html
Also, always check with your doctor to see if there is a generic option. Keep in mind that although they are the same drug, they are not exactly the same and your system may react differently depending on the manufacture, dose and how the medication is released into your system. Also, if you obtain pharmaceuticals through the mail, they may not be the real deal. Be cautious.

If you qualify for Medicare, you may want to check into *Qualified Medicare Beneficiary Program* (QMB). This is a Medicaid program to assist you with paying for Medicare. You can only have a very minimal income and no assets to qualify but it is worth looking into if you are in that situation.
https://www.medicaid.gov/medicaid/prescription-drugs/index.html

It is worth mentioning that in addition to assistance financially, you may want to assess if all the drugs are necessary or if you could alter your lifestyle and "wean" off of some medications. Keep in mind that everything you put in your body matters. It changes you, perhaps in small insignificant ways, but you can't really know the extent to which it will change you. This goes for supplements, herbs, vitamins, and all other non-prescription or over the counter products. You can research individually, does this product interact with other medications?

But if you take several medications, this can be a challenge. I wish there was a database/software that you could list everything taken and have it run a complete interaction profile but to my knowledge that doesn't exist. Just as with the Warfarin, even food can alter medications.

Don't assume that the medical professionals or even the pharmacist catches everything. My mother took Celebrex for years which apparently you are not supposed to do. Then she took Warfarin for several months before the thrombosis lab called and said for her to stop the Celebrex. (Increased potential of stomach bleed). Vitamins may seem innocent. We have all heard that you just pee out what your body doesn't need but that is not always the case. My partner's father had heard that Potassium pills were good for restless leg syndrome which he self- diagnosed himself to have. He also thought if one was good then several were better. He started suffering from an inability to walk and back pain. A trip to the doctor and X-rays didn't reveal anything other than the expected level of arthritis for someone in their 80's. He was prescribed Meloxicam which was no help. The difficulty walking necessitated a wheelchair and it really seemed as if he was on his way out. My partner suspected the potassium and questioned her mother. Apparently, he was taking at least 4 or 5 a day. An immediate stop was put to that and within a week he was walking again albeit a little rickety. Turns out that excess potassium (hyperkalemia) can cause fatigue, dizziness, numbness, muscle pains and cramps, heart palpations and even death. He is lucky he didn't have a heart attack. He would go on to live another 18 months.

A study in 2022 reported that 66% of the US population takes prescription drugs. 39% of seniors take five or more per day. Many drugs were never meant to be taken long term yet once people start taking them they end up taking them for years with no idea of what side effects they could be causing. A great example of this is anti-depressants. Unfortunately, just saying no to the drugs is also a problem. Stopping a drug can be next to impossible if not dangerous. They suggest you work with your doctor to wean off a drug as cold turkey can lead to difficult side effects or serious repercussions. The perception is that drugs like OxyContin are addictive and difficult to quit, but the truth is that many people are dependent on all types of drugs and when you discontinue them your body goes through some type of withdrawal. The Direct-to-Consumer advertising has led to an increase of prescription drug use and in many cases is "selling" people on a cure for a disease they might not even have. Celebrities are used in ads to make the drugs or tests seem even more innocent or acceptable than they should be. Listen to or read the little tag line at the end listing all the negative side effects or contraindications. Other than the US, New Zealand is the only other country that allows direct to consumer ads. Bottom line, some medications save lives, some do not. Do your research.

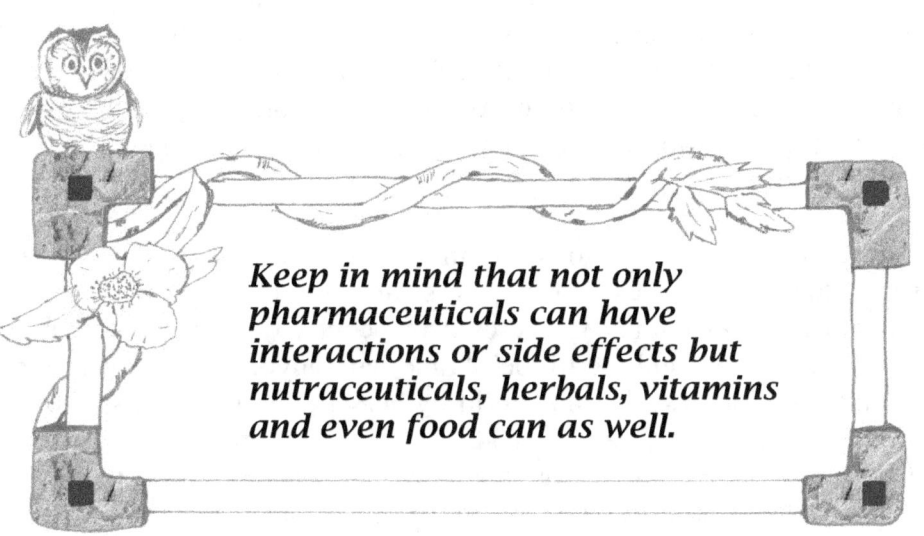

Keep in mind that not only pharmaceuticals can have interactions or side effects but nutraceuticals, herbals, vitamins and even food can as well.

Shoulder Pain

As previously explained, my mother had a shoulder replacement and despite the negative happenings afterwards, the procedure itself was successful. Now the other shoulder hurt. I enlisted the help of a friend who was a physical therapist to come to the house and come up with a routine of exercises that might help the shoulder from getting worse and perhaps strengthen her legs to assist with getting out of chairs. The therapist came for about six times but overall; it went over like lead balloons. I guess when you are done exercising you are done exercising. The more the shoulder hurt the more she didn't use it, so of course it "froze" making any movement very painful. Because of the aftermath of the previous shoulder surgery, we didn't think another shoulder replacement was a great idea.

There wasn't a cream we didn't try, or I should say that worked. I think it was three years of, "Can you put something on my arm"? At first that is an innocent request. After the 100 thousandth time, I couldn't help but grit my teeth at each request. In part because it was asked in a voice that you would expect someone pleading for their life might have and also because I knew it wasn't working. The placebo effect was in affect.

That voice. It wasn't the voice my mother used throughout our life; it wasn't the voice she used in business. She was a person that would have no problem talking to a crowd of people, walk into a CEO or VP's office, and stand toe to toe. Argue with anyone with a differing political opinion, traveled the world by herself, and now she spoke in almost a childlike manner and needed assistance with almost everything. Many times, Ron and I would look at each other and lament at the disappearance of the mother we knew. Ron had a difficult time with this and would often say something to her to get her mad because when she was mad, she would use her "old" voice that we were used to. I saw it differently. Life is a cycle, and it seems that if you make it to a ripe old age, not everyone, but many will become almost childlike with their emotions and need for care. This was our mother now; the one we remembered was gone and not coming back. In a way, I felt like every day I mourned that loss before the final loss.

Helping her get up out of chairs was a challenge because she didn't want the arm touched. In addition, because of her balance problem, being in front of her wasn't an option. The care centers use a belt device, similar to the one pictured here.

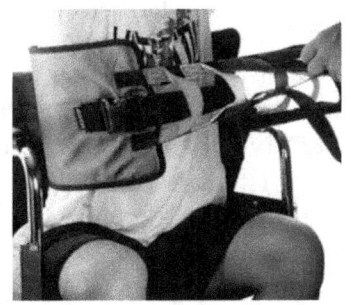

This is a great help for the caregiver's back if you can use it. I could not because there was no way she could move her arm to be out of the way and if I stood in front, she would resist coming towards me due to the balance issue. I had to work from the good arm side and pull her up by that arm. I got pretty good at it. It did help if she had shoes that would give her some traction. If they slipped, it would be a struggle. I used the same method getting her up out of the wheelchair or her rollator. And no, it wasn't great for my back.

Emergency Surgery

No, not for the shoulder. We were planning on going to lunch for Ron's birthday, but mom said she didn't feel well. Then it progressed to extreme pain in her mid-section. The Urgent care was closer, so we went there. That turned out to be a waste of time because we ended up with "We don't know" and a directive to the hospital. On the way there she threw up and continued to complain of extreme pain. Checking into an ER is always fun. Depending on the hospital that can take a bit of time. They did an X-ray/Scan. Turns out that her bowel was twisted in a couple of spots. Since we had the false alarm years ago during an ER visit, I did ask the surgeon's surety on this diagnosis and what would happen if surgery was not done. He said there was no question and that if surgery wasn't done immediately, first the bowel would die and then she would die a painful death. So, surgery. It is called a Volvulus when a loop of intestine twists around itself and the mesentery that supports it, resulting in a bowel obstruction. The surgery went well and because it was caught early enough, they were able to untangle things and no bowel needed to be removed. The after surgery was interesting.

When we met her after recovery, they were having trouble deciding what room she was going to, so we were sort of in the aisle way. She wasn't a person prone to swearing. In reply to how she was feeling, we got the following: "Shit, shit, shit, shit, oh, shit, shit, shit, etc." There would be a small break with silence and then the chant would begin again. Anyone who has interacted with someone after a surgery probably has funny stories. We laughed a bit. The next days were not as funny. She was trying to pull out her tubes, so I stayed with her throughout the night. When I went for a freshn' up break, the hospital had someone keeping an eye out and some family members were there as well. I got a call from Ron asking me to talk to her on the phone because she was convinced that the hospital workers asking her questions were really con artists and intended on going to her house to raid it while she wasn't there. I assured her no one was at the house and let her know I was on my way. Although, it could sometimes be a double-edged sword, I always felt grateful that she trusted me, and I could always calm her down. She said some other crazy things as well, but the next "issue" was that the nurses/doctor felt that she could be accumulating fluids in her stomach, and they did not want her to throw up. Their idea was to put a tube up her nose to drain it. It is called a nasogastric tube and it goes up the nose, down the esophagus and into the stomach. It can be used to remove or add fluids. I didn't see the first try but several family members did, it didn't go well. They tried putting the bed in an almost vertical position and tried it again. She screamed several times then pulled out what little progress they had made. We all requested that they stop. I don't think anyone has a fun time with that procedure unless they are unconscious. I have a feeling that the difficulty they were having was due, in part, to the numerous sinus surgeries that she had had. A couple of nieces were in the room during this and I think they were a bit traumatized. I have to admit, I was a bit as well. It is one thing to deal with your loved one that has pain but watching someone hurt them is another thing altogether.

The next day she was a bit better but still having effects from the surgery/anesthesia. She was in a bit of a foul mood but did offer up a great laugh for us albeit she was dead serious when she said, "Who is going to check me out of this dump?" It might be another one of those, "you had to be there" moments, but we all had a great laugh and even she thought it was funny when we told her about it months later. She was not doing well enough to go home but needed to leave the hospital, so she was sent to a care center.

Rehabilitation Center

It was just about a four-week stint. Clearly, she did not bounce back after this surgery. She may not have been great before, but now we slipped a big notch. She now needed assistance to walk to the bathroom. For the surgery they had to cut the abdominal wall, the scar was about five inches long, so I imagine that made things a little difficult, but she just seemed worse than she should have been. She didn't want to eat in the dining room. She did the rehab time they scheduled but not with a great attitude. The occupational therapist tried to get her to play games to assist with mental and physical rehab. She didn't play games on her best day so that was a waste of time, but it did show a vivid example of her decline.

Most nurses do the best they can with the difficult patients they endure day after day, and of course, they try to keep the patient calm and happy. Keep in mind my mother already complained of arm pain so when she is asked about her pain level, she tells them it is in the upper level. So, they gave her OxyCodone. For the first couple weeks she mostly slept, and we had to continually explain to her why she was there. I didn't expect her to get up and run circles around the room, but this just wasn't working. I asked them to please stop giving her Oxy. They supposedly noted it on her chart and for a couple of days she seemed to be doing better and was coming around at least mentally. At this time, I was still working at our recruiting business so I would go there in the mornings and visit with her in the afternoons at the care center. Here's a piece of advice that I was only so-so at. When your person is in the hospital or care center, take the opportunity for yourself to take a breather. There are professionals whose job it is to take care of your person. You will be back on duty soon enough. Recharge, if at all possible. Having said that, you do still need to stay on top of things and here is an example of why. After the few days of my mother doing better, I came in her room to find her just as incoherent and sleepy as she was before. I went to the nurse's station and asked if they had given her OxyCodone again. Yeah, the nurse said, "She complained of pain." I said, I specifically asked that she not be given it. "Oh," she said, "I didn't know." Call me silly but in an era where everything is documented electronically down to a single pill, is it too much to note the family's directives? Anyway, my point is that you need to keep track of what clinical people are doing and giving to your person just as a precaution, *don't assume anything*. That's a good life strategy anyway and one of the agreements in, **"The Four Agreements"** by Miguel Ruiz.

During this "rehab" it became obvious that walking had become more difficult for her. Her bedroom at home was up a very long flight of stairs which we were going to have to do something about anyway and now with the decreased mobility, we needed to make some changes before she came home. We did toss around the idea of the stair lift and although it was pricey it wasn't about that so much as that when she got to the top, she would have a difficult time getting out of the chair and that seemed a bit dangerous. We decided to clear out a room right as you enter the house that had been a reading room. We moved her bed, nightstand, and TV downstairs and fixed up the room to be a welcoming bedroom environment. The thought was it would be more convenient for her as it would be on the same floor as the kitchen (which at the time she was still frequenting on her own), she would have access to a bathroom, and she would be on the main level for family and friend visitors.

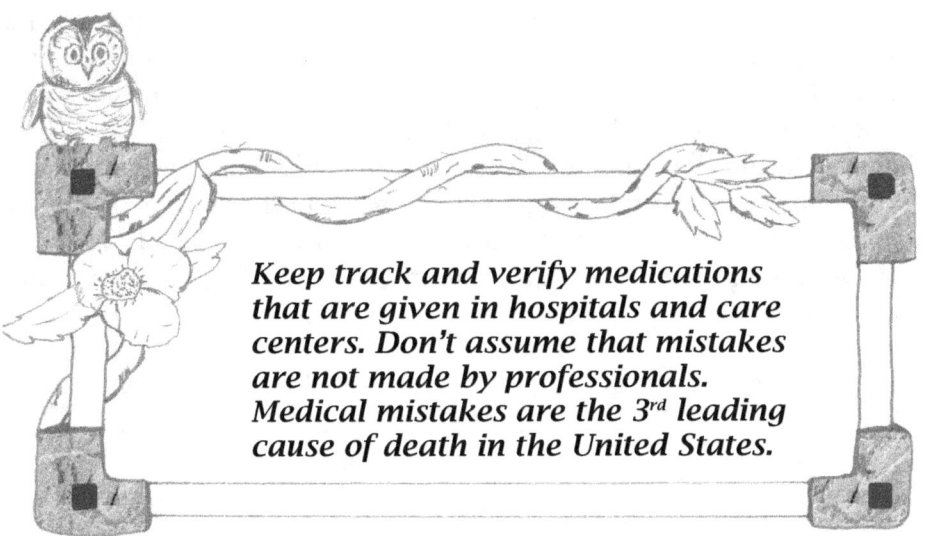

Keep track and verify medications that are given in hospitals and care centers. Don't assume that mistakes are not made by professionals. Medical mistakes are the 3rd leading cause of death in the United States.

Back Home

After about four weeks she came home. Mentally, she was doing better but walking was still a challenge, so I got her a walker. We already had a rollator for when we went places but, in my opinion, those are not as great for around the house. Both devices have a correct way of usage, but good luck if you can get your person to do so correctly. The tendency is to push the device well out in front with a hunched over posture. I am not sure why, but it is as if they resent the need for it and are trying to push it the hell out of their way. I don't know how many times I watched her get close to the bed and push the walker away when she still had four or five more feet to go to her destination. If they still have balance and only need it occasionally, that would be no big deal. But once they become dependent on it, that can be a problem. Although they may get to the destination fine, when they need to get up and go again, the device is not within reach.

The bedroom on the main floor did present a challenge. Although there was a bathroom, it did not have a shower. Getting her up a full flight of stairs wasn't an option. As I mentioned prior, she had a building next door for her office. It did have a shower on the ground level. There was still a stair hurdle albeit smaller than a full flight. The house entrance had four stairs. At this point she could slowly negotiate the stairs and get into a wheelchair waiting for her at the bottom. (Metal railings had already previously been installed.) I would wheel her over to the other building where she could get up two stairs and back into the wheelchair. I would roll into the bathroom and using the slick shower chair described on page 29 push her into the shower. It wasn't long before the stairs were too difficult. At that point I had the small portable ramps on the two-stair entrance and the large ramp on the main entrance.

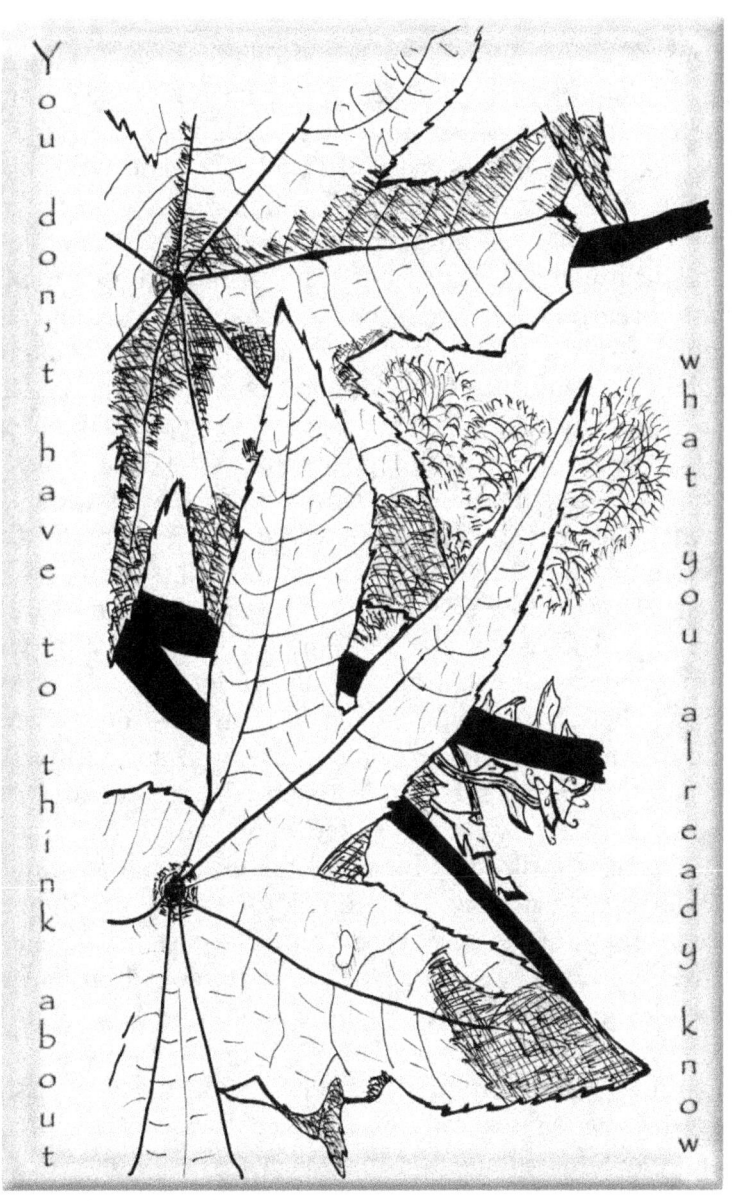

Shower Time

When my mother could still walk reasonably well, I only assisted her getting in and out of the shower so she felt safe (even with the bars), but she did her own wash up. Later, we got to the stage where the shower bench was necessary, and I had to do the wash up. The first time I thought it was awkward. You think of a shower as a time of solitude and privacy so although my mother never said so, I am sure she thought it just as awkward as I did. Although it certainly wasn't a common occurrence, I had seen her naked before, but still…. We developed a sort of ritual. If the weather was warm enough, I would wheelchair her out to the sun, get her a Diet Coke and install the foam curlers in her hair. To be clear, I have never operated curlers so there was a tiny learning curve. It happens that it makes a difference which way you roll. Despite the awkwardness of those first few times, there was something special about that whole process. Frequent reflections bring tears because I enjoyed that part of caring for her. Well, for the most part. Towards the end, I think it was just too hard for her. Crying takes it to a different level. I had already been assisting with shower time for about a year prior to the relocation of the bedroom. Previously, her shower was a walk-in in an on-suite to her bedroom. Despite me installing grab bars on the way in and in the shower, she still felt unsafe. Since she couldn't stand for any length of time, I put in a shower chair. The shower had about an 8" entry so I guess it wasn't exactly a walk-in and it was difficult for her to scale. We could have altered it but since she already needed assistance, we just powered through it. At this stage I mostly assisted with the in and out and toweling, not a big deal. Now as time moved on and the shower location changed, I needed to be more hands on.

I don't think seniors are any too happy about being naked. It's cold. Shower day, which was only once a week, was not her favorite. Also, keep in mind the shoulder/arm was a serious source of pain, and moving it to take shirts off and on was difficult. Once de-clothed, she would make the transition from wheelchair to shower chair, (pictured on page 29) and I could push her in. I had a removable shower head which I would have her hold while I soaped up the washcloth and washed everything but her personal areas. For that, I gave her the washcloth and let her do the honors. There were times that I felt like maybe I should intervene, but I didn't. I tried to put myself in her shower chair and I couldn't imagine anyone doing that for me.

After shower time, if the weather was warm enough, we would roll outside into the sun, or, if not, go inside and listen to an audible book while I rolled up her hair. This wasn't a previously shared mother and daughter type of interaction. The times in the shower when she complained or cried wasn't my favorite, but the hair rolling time I always felt that it was a special time that I would remember fondly in the future, and I was right.

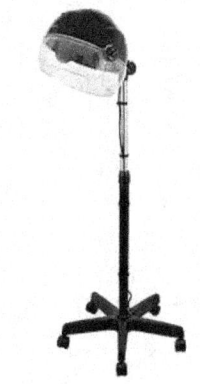

There might have been a lot of things that were not healthy about her, but hair wasn't one of them. She still had thick hair that took awhile to dry. Of course, I used a blow dryer, but it never seemed to dry it well enough. They make a home version of the dryers in the salons that worked well. It is a bit loud but did the job better than the handheld. Many different versions are available and will run you around $140. I also think it allowed her to reminisce about the beauty salon days of her past.

Her arm pain made it difficult to change in and out of clothes. Since she needed to be comfortable and the clothes couldn't have zippers or buttons, I came to the conclusion that jammies and everyday clothes were not that different. My solution was to buy stretchy pants or shorts and cotton tops from the second hand. In the morning was a new outfit which she wore all day and slept in. The next day was a new outfit. I ended up doing a lot of laundry and it does wear out the clothes quickly but since they were bought at a very low price, I just tossed them at a certain point and bought more. Despite the fact that she would never have entered a second hand store on her own, she did like the fun styles I bought and always having something new, well new to her.

Chapter Seven

Senior Care Suggestions

Some things we just take for granted. In addition to gravity and waking up each morning, we expect to be able to always do the little things, like clip our toenails. Unfortunately, a lot of things become difficult. If you are caring for a senior, in addition to Mani-Pedis, you might want to consider some other little changes that might make a big difference.

Jars and lids are difficult to remove. There are many aids you can buy to help with this but if they don't work, you might want to consider putting things in containers that are easy to open and well-marked. Keep this in mind if you are doing the shopping. My mom preferred the little 8oz bottled Diet Cokes because she could open them herself and easily hold them in her hand. I purchased little individual two-cookie packs, single serving cheese, etc. Easy for her to get herself. The smaller versions or individual packages are more expensive, but they are worth it.

Stuff is hard to reach. Consider a kitchen remodel. Move the things that are most utilized in the middle cabinetry. Standing on step stools or getting on the floor could be a challenge or possibly a really bad event. Cleaning the house will at some point become too difficult. If you have help or can hire someone to clean that is great, but occasionally you should be the one to do so. This will allow you to see what changes might need to be made or to see more accurately how your person is living day to day, what tasks may pose a challenge, or perhaps items that should be removed from the house.

Hygiene

Don't assume that they have it covered. You may need to assist with more than just nails, hair washing for instance. They make a "dry" shampoo that goes on like a mousse and doesn't need to be rinsed. It does make the hair a bit fresher but obviously doesn't clean the hair or scalp. Even just a tub of water and a tiny amount of shampoo and some towels could be enough tools to keep hair reasonably clean. As mentioned before, baths and showers become very challenging if not impossible.

Depends

Despite the youngish people in the commercials modeling their stylish disposable underwear, no one wants to need these. Honestly, I think it does help that they try to make them stylish. My mother probably started wearing them about four years prior to her death. Accidents happen and it is much easier to toss them and get a new pair than to constantly clean. I know it isn't ecologically friendly and we are spoiled in our current society but that is just one easy fix that makes life a little less stressful for the caregiver and the person in that unfortunate situation.

Handicapped Parking

If you are the taxi for anyone with difficulties walking, you can ask their doctor for a letter requesting a handicapped placard you can hang in your car. It allows you to park close and just as important it is really helpful to have the extra space to maneuver the wheelchair and patient. You will need to get the placard from your DMV.

Helpful Book

Every state has its own ***"Senior Blue Book"***. This contains helpful articles, businesses, and resources centered around senior living or caring for seniors. They are typically found at the entrances of grocery or drug stores.

Clutter

I mentioned this earlier, but it is worth repeating. If someone finds it difficult to get around with or without mobility devices, clutter can be an accident waiting to happen. Recently, I went to the house of a gentleman in his 90's that had just recovered from a broken leg caused by a throw rug in the middle of the kitchen floor. He used a rollator to get around primarily to steady himself, not surprisingly, he was afraid of falling. His family had so much crap on the floor of the hallways that he had to lift his rollator up and scrunch the wheels closer together to get to the next room. Did they want him to fall again? And yes, there were still a couple of throw rugs as well as a towel on the floor of the bathroom. Just because you can see or dodge obstacles doesn't mean everyone can. Clear paths are essential.

Gadgets & Gizmos

There were a few inexpensive gadgets that came in quite handy. My mother had a period when she was prescribed oxygen, and an oxygenator was delivered so that no tanks were needed. She wasn't very thrilled about wearing the tubing and would often remove it. I needed to make sure her oxygen wasn't dropping too low, so I got a Pulse Oximeter which shows the blood oxygen level and the heart rate.

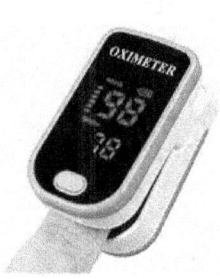

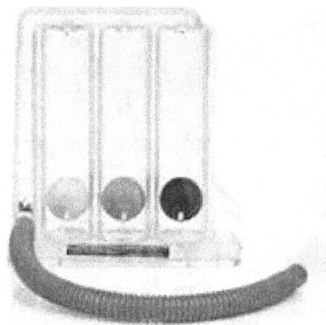

Again, because of the low oxygen levels, I got a Spirometer which shows the volume of air that the person can blow and **if** they will use it several times a day can help increase their ability to breath.

I called it the easy button, a little device meant for the blind. When you press it, it gives the time and day of the week. My mother could not see clocks anymore, but the real value was to reorientate her. Since sleeping increased and was throughout the day, it became difficult for her to know what time it was. Many times, my mother would wake up at two in the morning thinking it was time to start the day. This really helps.

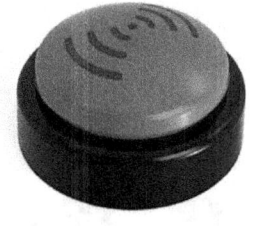

I hesitate to suggest something electronic in nature since it will be obsolete by the time I finish writing the sentence, but...I had concerns when I went home at night that my mother could have a problem and would need to get in touch with me. Early on she could just use the phone. But even with a large button phone, at a certain point that didn't work. I didn't want a sophisticated system for a monthly fee so I purchased one on Amazon that I thought would work. Like everything, there are a lot of choices. The one I got allowed you to program telephone numbers. It had a little amulet-like device that could be worn around the neck (she wouldn't), so I attached it to her walker figuring she would likely be near that no matter what had happened. It would call what number was programmed in first. If no one answered or a voice mail picked up, it would automatically call the 2nd number programed, then the 3rd, or 911 if you wanted that as a choice. Once the connection was made, you could converse back and forth just as if both parties were using phones. The first time she used it, she was pretty upset and confused but it allowed me to let her know I was on my way. She only used it a few times but when I was called at 5am, rushed over and stabilized the situation, went back home, and was called again at 8am, I knew that my decision to move into her house was made.

Depending on what company you go with and what you need it to do, you could be looking at $100-300.

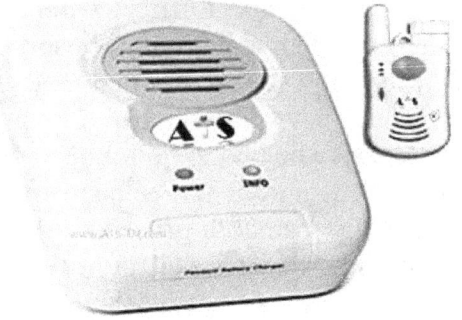

Going Places

The wheelchair was a necessity when we went out. Knowing how difficult it was for my mother to be "captive" in her own home, I always tried to take her anywhere she wanted to go. Some of these were simple, like going for a burger and shake. Some were events that she used to do in the past and didn't want to give up, like festivals or concerts. Those were typically a logistical nightmare, and we would have struggles with parking or the bathroom or such. Many times, she would be upset about something during the outing and complain or even cry but when we arrived home or the next day she would say, "That was fun wasn't it?" Huh? Despite that, I continued to keep up the outings until it really just became too difficult. I think when you get older, you still remember the activity as it was or how it felt when you were younger and unfortunately most things really just are not how you remembered or in many cases, the activity really isn't fun anymore. I have gone to numerous rock concerts starting from about age 10. The last couple I went to were disappointing on multiple levels. Now I prefer to buy a concert DVD and park myself on the couch. The drinks are much cheaper and there is no line at the potty. Things change.

So, we limited the fun outings. Another outing that proved to be a nightmare was to the doctor's office. After the volvulus surgery, she was still in the care center when the hospital/doctor wanted to do a follow up office visit. They transported us there, but she was really in no state to deal with any of it. We had a long wait which she wasn't a fan of on a good day. She had to go to the bathroom and although I did manage the two of us and the wheelchair in a bathroom or stall, let's just say, it was never a smooth procedure. I am not sure which one of us was more stressed, but it wasn't a good time. Previously, doctors' visits had been difficult but not on that scale. I was able to reduce a few visits by getting her primary care doctor to refill her prescriptions by email request. Now that telemedicine is gaining ground, this might not be as much of a concern.

Pain, Pain, and More Pain

My mother had a bad knee which was painful for her all her life and made it difficult to get around as she aged. In her early 20's she was just walking along when her kneecap shattered. In the 1950's treatment was limited but they were able to put in an artificial kneecap. As a result of this previous surgery, she was not a candidate for a knee replacement even if she was strong enough to endure it. We tried an expensive brace from Don Joy which turned out to be a waste of time. Maybe a little too late to try this apparatus. It was specially fitted and looked similar to the one shown here. It was a challenge to get on and stay in position and because her knee curved in towards the other knee, the added material from the brace made it so that her knees rubbed together when she walked. That was a short-term product for us.

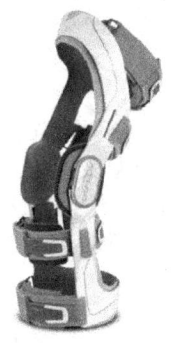

We tried injections with cortisone, Synvisc, and Zilretta (extended-release steroid injection). Nothing helped. At this point we realized that we were out of options for the knee. The thing was that even though the knee was painful, the shoulder was where she was having the most difficulty. We also tried cortisone and Synvisc injections for the shoulder, no help. We utilized every cream/patch, capsaicin, Diclofenac gel (Voltarern), Lidocaine (Salon Pas, Lidoderm), Menthal (Icy Hot), Salicylates (Aspercream), Doterra's Deep Blue, THC/CBD creams, etc. For about two years, several times a day, I was asked, "Can you put something on my arm?" I continued to put stuff on her arm even though I was pretty sure it made no difference, but as I mentioned before, the placebo effect I think is very real and it made her feel like something was being done. In her last few weeks, she stopped asking.

In addition to creams and patches, she took a few over the counter Tylenol every day and two of the nighttime pills. She had also been prescribed Tramadol. Since she still complained of pain, I wasn't sure how much the drugs were helping, if at all. Pain is a touchy subject. It is subjective and no one can know what you are experiencing. Obviously, pain medication addiction is a huge issue, and we have all heard the negative about OxyContin. I really struggled with this topic.

When Hospice came in (more on that later), in addition to Tramadol, they prescribed Morphine. My mother was already experiencing dementia symptoms and my internal question was how much was happening regardless and how much confusion was being caused by the drugs? I didn't want her to be so out of it that she couldn't communicate, yet she still complained of pain. Hospice explained that there wasn't a possibility of addiction at this stage, and I shouldn't be worried about giving her more medication. Still, it was difficult to be the decider on this topic.

A friend of mine's husband had been taking a fair bit of Oxy for several years. In retrospect she could see that he had signs of dementia, but she had written it off as drug side effects. Nothing she could have done about it anyway but just an example of the difficulty in doling out pain med for others.

The Bitch Named Dementia

No one wants a visit from this bitch. Although the Egyptians documented the concept as early as 2000 BC, the term was coined in 1797 and is from the Latin, meaning, "being out of one's mind." It is now used as an umbrella term for cognitive impairment. There are several types of dementia, including the dreaded Alzheimer's. I think everyone worries about themselves when they start to forget things which could be a sign, but is more likely that we have too much chatter in our heads. More than once I have found myself starting to put the crackers in the fridge and thought, "Oh my god, I am losing it."

In my mother's case, it seemed to sneak up gradually and then accelerated with the last surgery really moving the needle. In retrospect, she had several of the "signs" about four or five years prior, some of which included difficulty managing money, mood swings, avoiding company, confusion, being unmotivated, misplacing objects or putting them in unusual places (like crackers in the fridge), or used tissues in a drawer, problems finding the right words, poor short-term memory, trouble concentrating or thinking, and trouble completing mundane tasks.

As I mentioned, I was really concerned that the drugs might be making the dementia worse or at least the confusion worse but what are the options? Seeing your parent slowly become dependent is really tough. Seeing them in pain, tough. Helping them with physical hurdles, tough. Watching them lose their mind is just heart wrenching. A neighbor of my mother's who came to visit regularly had both parents develop Alzheimer's at the same time. That falls under my motto: "It can always get worse." I can't even imagine that situation. As hard as it was to care for my mother, at least she knew who I was. Also, she never got violent or hateful to me which I know happens with many seniors and their caregivers.

So, then one day we went from normal confusion to hallucinations. Seeing people who were not there, saying things like, "I just got back from the post office," despite the fact she hadn't left the house recently or done those type errands for at least three years. Although we eventually did get to this stage, at this point it turned out that she had a urinary tract infection (UTI). This is very common and often is not diagnosed because the odd behavior is written off as dementia. Also, one typically assumes that a UTI would announce itself with pain while urinating, but that is not always the case with seniors. They treat it with antibiotics which in this case came with similar side effects, as in more hallucinations. The doctor insisted that antibiotics wouldn't do that, but I have talked to several people that experienced the same negative symptoms and have since read some doctors reporting that hallucinations are indeed a real side effect and often misdiagnosed in seniors as Sundowners Syndrome. Sundowners Syndrome, or sundowning, is a state of confusion that occurs later in the afternoon and into the night. This state of confusion is most often found in patients who have dementia and is comprised of a range of behaviors, including increased confusion, anxiety, and aggression. Sometimes people with this condition tend to pace or wander, and they may ignore or not hear instructions.

Although UTIs are more common in women, a friend of mine's husband was experiencing angry, accusatory, outbursts and was undiagnosed for over a week before finally identifying the UTI. Although he was treated for it, his system was ultimately not able to rebound, and he ended up passing away. It just seems to me that it would make sense to jump to the UTI conclusion first and rule it out since it is so common. This again goes to my previous statement about taking charge of the situation and not waiting for the medical professionals to get to the answer. Don't assume they have everything under control.

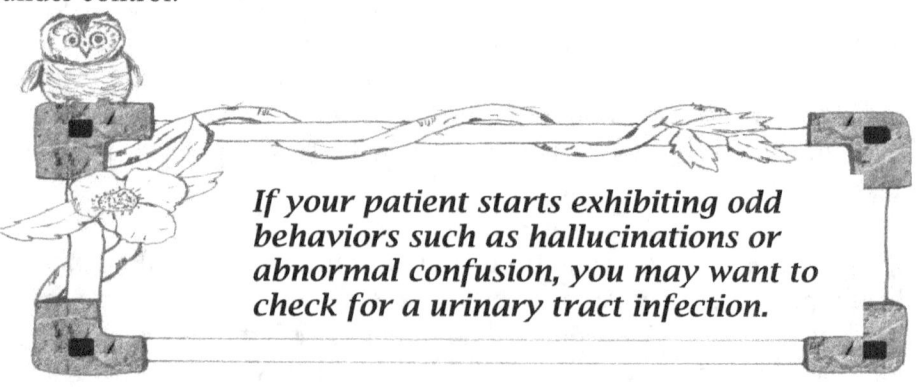

If your patient starts exhibiting odd behaviors such as hallucinations or abnormal confusion, you may want to check for a urinary tract infection.

Bringing in Hospice

I talked about this earlier in regard to Ron. It made sense to bring in hospice because I knew he had a short time to live, that it would get ugly, and I would need help if for no other reason than to supply the morphine. In my mother's case, it wasn't so obvious. My mother had what the industry refers to as the "dwindles," meaning a slow decline but nothing severe or immediately life threatening.

You will want to think this one thorough before engaging hospice if your person is not imminent. What you are agreeing to when taking this step is that you are no longer going to seek hospital treatment, in other words, you are going to let things "dwindle" and not utilize any life saving measures. Let's say your person is having a heart attack. You can absolutely change your mind, call 911 and have them rushed to the hospital. That would cancel the hospice service. Later, you might really need what hospice offers, so you can see why you can't jump back and forth.

There is another reason why not to call hospice. If you are looking for answers, how long does my person have, what or how will things happen, or if you are expecting help with the day to day, you would be better off calling Ghostbusters, because hospice won't be a help.

Here's what hospice does offer. As a part of the beginning process, they have a nurse come out for an evaluation. There is a doctor on staff that they confer with but who does not make a visit. They have a social worker and chaplin that pay you a visit. Perhaps you have that need. I didn't and neither my mother or Ron would even speak to them. Depending on the "needs" of the patient, they decide on the frequency of nurse visits and the nurse may not always remain the same). In my mother's case, they started with once every two weeks. They have a CNA that can come out once a week to assist with hygiene. You might find this to be very helpful. In my case, while the CNA was trying to do her job, my mother kept yelling for me to come into the bathroom, so, not a break for me after all. Easier to do it myself.

One of the "offers" they had was to have a volunteer sit with her for an hour. Great. First, I would need to explain to my mother that I was leaving her with a stranger for an hour, then I could jump in my car, race to the Barnes & Noble, scan a few books, suck down a coffee and rush back. Never mind. There were a few neighbors who offered and maybe I should have taken them up on it earlier in the game, but once you are consumed by the caretaking monster, unplugging is just difficult.

Medicare pays for Hospice so nothing they did came out of our pocket but when I saw what they were charging Medicare, I got a bit upset. For the two nurse visits, a couple of CNA visits, and some supplies, it was almost $5000/month. Whaaat? For half of that I could have hired a personal nurse to come on a regular basis, establishing a rapport where I could trust leaving for a bit and my mother could perhaps bond. But they don't pay for that type of care and unfortunately, we didn't have the finances to do so.

In my case, the "value" to me was that I didn't have to worry about taking her to the doctor when there was a problem, like the UTI and medications being altered as needed. In regard to medications, Hospice will take over the ordering of most medications that the person has been taking. In my mother's case, she was taking Eliquis, and anticoagulants were not ordered by them as they are considered more of a life-saving medication. Towards the end we agreed that there wasn't a need to continue that medication anyway. I had also stopped bothering with vitamins. She was having difficulty swallowing them. There was an incident where one got lodged in her throat. It was scary for me but traumatized her. I could have gotten liquid vitamins but again, what would be the point? Vitamins are not going to change anything at this point in life. In fact, Ron used to give her grief about her Diet Cokes. "You know they are not good for you." If you make it to your 80's, toss the rules, do whatever brings a smile to your face. Ultimately, she did not die from too much Diet Coke.

Anyway, I think hospice is a good idea for the very end, but you have to decide if it is any benefit early on. If you have help, siblings or other family members, you may be able to get by without them. No matter how great the Hospice company is, they are not likely to do the job like you do or would like them to do.

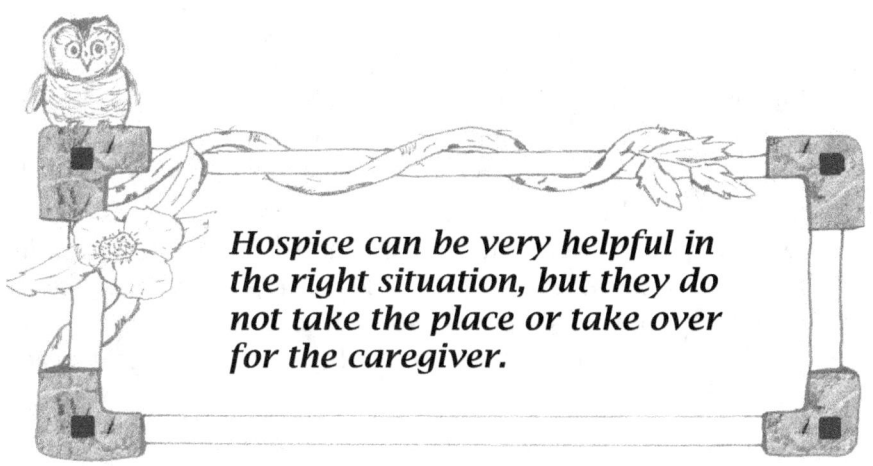

Hospice can be very helpful in the right situation, but they do not take the place or take over for the caregiver.

More Than One Caregiver

My experience is from the perspective of the person in charge. Although my remaining brother helped some evenings and weekends, he still deferred to me for guidance. I read a book on a caregiver's experience where she had been the sole caregiver for several years, giving up her career to do so. Then a couple of siblings came in, didn't like how she was doing things, and didn't agree on the father's future medical treatment. They were able to get a court order and essentially stripped her of her caregiving power. All I have to say is that I am grateful my brother wasn't like that, or I might have been locked away for seriously injuring my sibling. I believe I mentioned earlier about the possessiveness that occurs over your "patient." I only bring this example up because I think it is important if there is going to be more than one cook in the kitchen that you establish early on who is the head chef and who are the sous chefs and what your expectations are down to the very end. This part of life is emotional enough without fighting about it or perhaps losing your ability to be a part of decisions for your loved one.

Partners

If it is your partner you are taking care of, you are likely an island of one. A friend of mine was taking care of her husband at the same time as I was my mother, and we had a lot of similar challenges, but I always felt like her situation was worse. I got to go home (initially), and she was there 24-7. Not to mention, the difference between potentially losing a parent whom we all expect to lose at some point and losing your best friend or soul mate that you pictured growing old together with. But if it isn't your partner you are caring for, how does this person fit in with your caregiving obligations?

Long story, but my partner wasn't able to assist me in any direct capacity. Moral support once home or holding down the fort was very helpful to me, but everyone has a threshold for patience and understanding. If you don't exceed your partner's threshold, you will be doing well. No one can really know you or what goes through your head on a normal day, but certainly, no one understands the emotions, stress, and total consumption that caregiving becomes unless they have experienced it themselves and even at that, everyone will process their situations differently.

My partner didn't understand why I just didn't get others to fill in for me. As I mentioned before, I should have done that earlier on, but I would say even the last couple of years, even if I physically took time away, I would have taken IT with me anyway. I thought I was handling things pretty well. Certainly, I admitted I was stressed but I was doing it. I hadn't gotten in the car and driven to the end of the earth or any such thing. People often asked, "How are YOU doing?" Of course, they often asked that in front of my mother. Not sure what they expected me to answer. As far as my mother was concerned, I was great and happy to be there. But really, it was tough at times. My partner felt like I had that wild-eyed-edge-on-a-precipice-look. I didn't think so but one day I took a real look at my friend who was taking care of her husband and I saw that look. Ok, so I probably had it too. Honestly, I am not sure how I could have done differently, but I should have figured out a way to not push my partner to the side while I mired myself in the care of others. Although I did think I handled things as well as I could, I did eventually have a meltdown, albeit a small one.

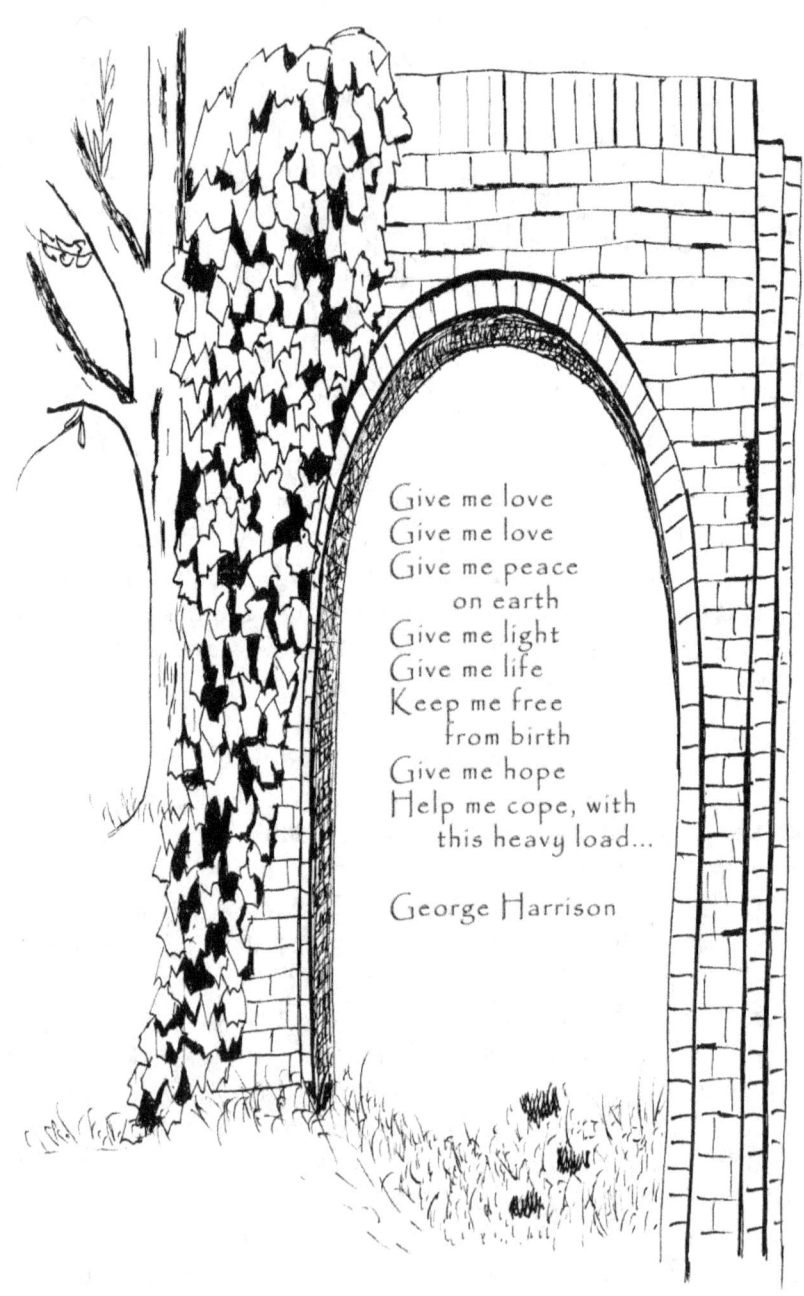

Chapter Eight

Burnout

After Ron became ill, upon arriving at my mother's house, I would pause before opening the door. I would wonder what would be greeting me on the other side. What state would they be in or is today the day I would find someone dead. The constant stress of being responsible for someone's everything is overwhelming. It surprised me that I could spend the whole day doing just that. How is it possible that it could take that much time and energy to take care of one person? People would say, "I bet you have burn out" and I would reply, no, burnout happened a long time ago.

Planning meals was always challenging. Coming up with different ideas especially when I had two picky eaters to deal with was difficult. I would ask them to please help me with suggestions. Rarely did I get any input. One day after what I made wasn't met with overwhelming enthusiasm, I had a little flair up. "Why don't you both get your own damn dinner." I got over myself and continued business as usual, but sometimes I found it very difficult to not get frustrated and lose my normal cheery disposition. I am sure there were many times when even though I was trying to be accommodating, my facial expressions betrayed me.

I think it was about October when I started to live at my mother's full time. Fortunately, as I have said, I still had one remaining brother and he came in for me a couple evenings and a weekend day so I could go home for a few hours, visit with my partner, pet my dog, then turn around and come back. In some ways this was more difficult than if I were in another state and couldn't get home easily.

Mom had been slipping further into dementia land. Although my brother was very capable and did a great job with her, she still wanted me to always be there. Many evenings when I got there she would be in a very agitated state. In this dementia state of mind, she was at the mall, the bank, a care center, a hotel but not in her room. It took a bit of persuading to convince her that it was indeed her bed, her room, and her house that she was in. Once she told my brother that I had kidnapped her and wouldn't let her go home. Although the trip to the bathroom was a very common event and literally fifteen feet from her bed, she would ask, "Where is the bathroom here?" I must admit there were times when my brother and I would have a laugh about something she said or thought she was doing, but it really was such a heartache for me that she was going through this.

I had a routine that worked well during the day, but it was very challenging at night. Because she was getting confused and agitated, hospice prescribed Lorazepam in a cream form which I would rub on the inside of her wrist. I think it helped a bit. A dose of morphine was given close to 10pm, as well as a dose of Melatonin. I would always make sure she went to the bathroom around 11pm. I slept on the couch. If I got up and looked over the back, I could see her in her bed just in the next room. Most of the time I slept with one eye open or at least listening to every sound. Some nights we made it to about 1am before I heard her getting up and heading to the bathroom. Initially, I only got up if she was gone for a long time or struggled to get back into bed. It wasn't long before every trip was a struggle. Then it repeated at 3am, 4:30am, 6am. Sometimes it would start at 1130pm. I'd say, "What you doing?" She would say, "I have to go to the bathroom." "You just went 30 minutes ago." "I don't care, if I got to go, I got to go." It was so random. There were nights where it was only once or twice and she slept most of the day; there were nights when she was up every hour and awake most of the day. Hospice did change the dosage, but it really didn't make much difference. I just kept thinking, I am so exhausted, how can this 84-year-old person taking that amount of drugs keep getting up throughout the night? It wasn't always to the bathroom. A few times she was in the kitchen. "What ya doing?" "I need to find my luggage." The luggage-trip-hotel theme happened several times. I am sure I overthought this, but I wondered, in some crazy way, was she preparing for her final trip? I would imagine it was that she loved to travel so thinking she was vacationing was a lot better than being trapped in your bedroom for months.

Sometimes I could go back to sleep, sometimes not. It didn't much matter because the sleep was only fleeting anyway. I was so tired, so stressed. I wasn't sure how long I could keep this up. I already felt my life was on hold, and I had no problem with that if we were talking months, but what if this could go on for years? I have to be honest, there were times that I wished she would have a heart attack and go in her sleep, partly because I was so fried and partly because it was already so hard to watch her decline, I just couldn't imagine how much worse it could get. Thinking that I would actually wish her to have a heart attack was also emotionally difficult. What did that say about me? I have a feeling I am not alone in this caretaking dichotomy.

Hospice can offer you a three-day break by taking the person to a facility. I thought about it, but the social worker advised me that sometimes dementia or confusion gets worse when they are removed from the home like that. Well, that certainly wasn't an option.

Christmas happened. Although I love the time of year, this one was the crappiest one in my record books. Stress was at an all time high at my home, dementia at an all time high for my mother, and no light at the end of the tunnel. The nurse came for her weekly visit and made the mistake of asking me how I was. (This was not in front of my mother) I really really hate to cry in front of people, but I couldn't not cry, and I needed her to tell me in her professional opinion what amount of time my mother had left. She of course couldn't give me any definitive answer, but she did think it was reasonably close. The human body is unpredictable. When we went back into the room with my mother, the nurse talked to her for a bit and in that discussion mentioned that she was dying. It was as if the thought had never occurred to her. Although her quality of life at this point was very poor, I still had a tinge of guilt at the seemingly blunt news from the nurse as it appeared to really devastate her. My mom said, "I'm dying?" The nurse said, something to the effect, "Well, you are winding down and in the final stages of life." My mother was a fighter, she was determined to persevere no matter what difficulties came her way, and now that this thought entered her mind, either she gave up because she really was tired of it all or because hope was now gone.

Empathy vs' Compassion

Although both terms are used interchangeably, they are very different emotions. Empathy literally means, in-suffering. So, while empathetic feelings are great initially as it can make us more aware of other's pain or misfortune, it is not good long term as you can experience distress and negative emotions thereby making two people miserable rather than helping anyone. "You cannot strengthen the weak by weakening the strong." Scientifically, it has been shown that the neurons in one person's brain can mirror another's. For example, one person could be in pain and the other person 's neurons are altered in the same manner despite not actually perceiving pain. Once we are overloaded with negative energy and stress, the amygdala hijacks our executive functions. Learning center, memory, decisions, all become compromised. I remember several times, even though, I thought I had my stuff together, doing really stupid things like leaving the stove on, forgetting appointments, and forgetting words or people's names. It makes sense now because I was clearly being too empathetic with my family. It is almost like you put yourself in their shoes which ultimately leads to emotional exhaustion.

So how is compassion different? Compassion means to have sorrow for the distress of others. It is a concern for other's wellbeing which elicits positive energy rather than the negative that empathy can have. You don't join them in their misery; you become the light to guide them. I read one of Cesar Millan's books regarding dog parenting. He talked about calm assertive energy making a difference in how the dog responded to commands. I am hopeful that my next fur child will have the benefit of me being calm and assertive because previous animals got the stressed overprotective version of me. Anyway, as I read that I wished I had the foresight to have calm energy while caring for my mother. Perhaps it would have helped her feel calmer. Who knows? I just know I was occasionally calm but more often the stressed-out overprotective version of me.

Final Days

During the day there was quite a bit of sleeping, and I would sit in her room and watch her. Many times, she would have what appeared to be really bad dreams, lots of twitching, odd sounds, etc. Evenings were the same as I mentioned earlier. Each day got progressively worse. A new difficulty arose. Whereas previously the short trip to the bathroom was an event, now it was almost impossible. I had a potty chair by the side of the bed which she rarely would use. Many times, she had no choice because she was just too weak, and her knee hurt too bad to make it to the bathroom. Her eating drastically reduced. Things that she normally had interest in were no longer of interest, chocolate, Diet Coke, most foods, Audible books, Fox News, etc. She was no longer asking me to put anything on her arm.

Death is going to happen when and how it is going to, and there isn't much we can do about it. But I think in some cases things get really bad so that parting with a loved one or telling them it is ok to go, is somehow easier because the alternative of continuing to watch them suffer just doesn't seem like a choice. The mother I grew up with, that person was already gone. This person was different, and I loved her, and now we were very close to this frail lady going as well.

Once she started to decline, the nurse visits increased. The bed we had made it too difficult for them to get on either side, so they insisted on bringing in a hospital bed. It had an air mattress that is hooked up to air so that it helps with reducing bed sores which amazingly she never got. (Ron did). The bed was far less comfortable than the one she had been used to. I did add a sheet of memory foam which helped a little. Here is one thing I absolutely wish I hadn't done. Because she couldn't get to the bathroom, I thought a catheter was the way to go. The nurse came out to insert the catheter which didn't seem at all pleasant but worse than that, it became infected. I will save you the description of that. I will just say that I wish I would have figured out the diapers and not put her through that or me for that matter. You can't unsee things.

I knew she was really close to not being able to communicate. Most of the neighbors and friends had routinely dropped by for a visit. I made sure to reach out to anyone that hadn't so that they could have some time with her. She had an out-of-state friend that I called for her. It was really a one-way conversation with her friend doing the talking but she was able to get out an "I love you." That was another tough moment for me as well as for her friend. Unfortunately, at this end stage, no discussions take place so I will say again, if you or anyone really want to "talk," it needs to be well before this stage.

Eating had stopped, not much drinking, drugs continued. She was awake but not very responsive. Hospice gave me a guide, *"The Eleventh Hour" by Barbara Karnes*. It detailed the signs of approaching death. There was also some literature with the hospice packet that broke down signs, last months, last weeks, last days. Between the two information sources it seemed that we were within hours so the whole family arrived in the evening. Several times her breathing was such that we thought it would be within minutes. I mentioned the death rattle previously in regards to Ron, a kind of gurgling sound that you may hear when people are dying. It happens because they are no longer able to swallow or cough, so saliva builds up in the back of the throat and upper airways. The fluid causes the rattling sound when air passes through. Both Ron and my mother had this to some degree, but it wasn't all the time and it doesn't mean they are ready to go at any moment. It can go on for quite a while. Hospice will give you drugs to assist with excess mucus, as well as a device to help remove it from the nose.

We all took time, talking to her, holding hands, letting her know we loved her, etc. When 11pm rolled around and she was at the same level, the family left for the evening. A few days earlier, one of the nurses had said to me, "Don't worry if you are not there when she passes, sometimes people prefer to be by themselves when they go". I was mentally and physically exhausted from all that had transpired in the past, but the final week was A LOT. Emotionally, the last evening with the family was spent on the roller coaster of death and dying. I went to sleep for a couple of hours.

The End

I knew she was dead. It was about 2am. She had been breathing so slight and hadn't moved in a couple of days, so I wasn't sure. I didn't hear a heartbeat, but I thought, maybe it is just faint. I lightly pounded on her chest which of course I had never done before so I am not sure what I expected there. I will say, however, and it could have been my imagination given that it was 2am and I wasn't in a great frame of mind, but the sound seemed hollow.

Nothing was as I expected. Maybe it was watching too many movies that I expected to be holding her hand and her last words would be, "I love you," then she would close her eyes and be gone. I had been so emotionally taxed for so long that I would have expected some moderate relief that she was free from her hell and me from mine, but neither of those things happened.

I waited until normal morning hours to call the nurse, and she came within a short time to "prepare" the body. The family all came to say their goodbyes before the mortuary came to pick her up. We watched as they shifted her from the bed to the stretcher and I don't know about anyone else but the sound and the visual of her body sort of dropping from one surface to the other seemed to me again, empty, hollow, like an inanimate object. Hard to forget this feeling/experience.

The next time we saw her was in the coffin, in the church complete with her bright red lipstick which I specifically asked them not to do. It was also slightly outside of lip boundaries. I get that based on the state of the body and time passed that decorating dead people is difficult, but it bothered me so much that I had to blot some of it off, which I must say was an extremely strange feeling.

The hospice company continued to send me letters for the first year offering counseling if needed. It said things like, "It is ok to be sad." Really? Too helpful. Anyway, they are there for talking if you need it. I have spoken about my mother/feelings to friends randomly as I am moved to do so, but really time is your friend and eventually it doesn't seem quite so painful or surreal. I am aware that many people are very emotional and painfully affected at all the anniversaries, birthdays, death days, holidays, etc. I don't find a particular need to be extra sad on special occasions. At first I had a lot of "flashbacks" of the last days and months which I thought would never go away. They haven't completely gone but they are slightly faded. I try to focus on the fun stuff from the past and not the last days, cause those just were not that great to remember.

Life must go on....

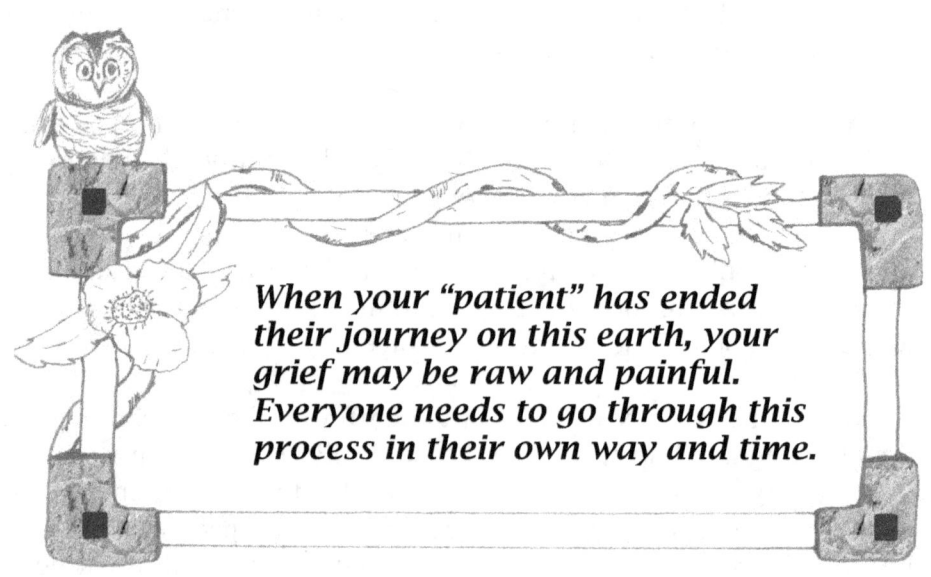

When your "patient" has ended their journey on this earth, your grief may be raw and painful. Everyone needs to go through this process in their own way and time.

Logistics

So many things to do and you are not likely to want to do any of it. I guess in some ways the to do list keeps you from melting down as much. Depending on your person's wishes, you might need to decide about donations. My partner's father was 86 and we didn't think that donation was a possibility but they wanted his eyes. This decision happens very soon after death and before the mortuary takes control. The mortuary handles the body with whatever path you are taking. They also get you the death certificates. The suggestion is to get six+ but I never used that many. The banks photocopied my original. I did mail a couple, but companies allow you to email an electronic copy, so I didn't need as many as I purchased.

If it is a spouse you have lost, and have accounts in both names, you will need to work on changing them to your name only. Consider bank, credit cards, titles, mortgages, utilities, etc. You may not want to change your bank account immediately if there is any possibility of receiving checks that would have both names listed. An often-overlooked and very tiny benefit for spouses is a $255 death benefit from social security. They call it a lump sum death payment (LSDP) and is available for the surviving spouse or child if either will be the recipient of the deceased persons social security benefits.

In our case, as mentioned previously, the house had a reverse mortgage which meant I had 90 days to show that it was for sale. This was challenging as the house and building next door were all full of stuff. I have seen examples where the family rents a dumpster, and everything gets tossed. I wasn't willing to do that. I had actually already been going through some of my mother's personal effects while I was staying there full time. There were a lot of items that really did belong in the trash. I set out with the same format as I had done with Ron's stuff (which I still had some of) and that was taking the things I wanted, ear-marking things that could have value to be sold and then allowing family to take what they wanted from what was left. Fortunately, I had a friend that had been doing well selling things on Facebook Marketplace, and he helped me list and sell quite a few items which took a lot of pressure off while I continued to go through the house. A few items were more suited to Ebay and I handled those.

I said earlier, "shit ain't worth shit," and it is true and surprising to me what we were and were not able to sell. My mother was an avid reader and had over 1,000 books. I offered them to neighbors and friends for free and I think I got four people to take maybe a total of 25 books. I should also mention this was the same time that COVID altered the universe, so a yard sale wasn't an option. She had several sets of Noritake china. The most I got was $100/set which was far less than the purchase price. Most of the furniture sold, piano, brass items, vases, live plants. Collectibles from travels like exotic masks did not sell. Like the books, my mother had an enormous amount of clothes. She had always dressed professionally and in designer fashions. No one wants those. Too dated for vintage clothing stores, sadly, it was all donated to a local charity. And I say sadly not because donating isn't a great idea, but my mother would have been devastated.

Several months prior someone had mentioned to my mother that kids throw away everything after their parents die, so she joked that I would do the same although I am not sure she was really joking. With the stuff that I mentioned, most can be sold, handed down, or donated. But not the personal items. Guess where the pictures and the journals ended up? A few years back, I had started to compile a life history for my mother editing her journals. I even read some journals as I went through the house. Unfortunately, they were so generic that even I had no interest in keeping them. She shared no emotions or thoughts about her life, only the facts, Ex: we saw this movie, I ate that, went here, etc. Albums and albums of pictures. Some family but many from travels which, unfortunately, she was only in a handful of. There were slides as well, and I viewed all those before tossing them. I did keep the old family pictures to pass down. I just mention this because it is a sad part of reality. When you die, with few exceptions, all that you did, worked on, or spent time on will be obviated.

It took me eight months to process everything and receive and accept an offer for the house. There was neither time nor money nor advantage to fixing the house in any way. The offer was based on an as is price.

It is funny but the last day in the house was nostalgic but not as sad as I thought. Our family had come and gone for 41 years. First the 'vibe" changed when Don died, then again with Ron, and drastically when my mother died. Then her things were removed from walls, floors, etc., and again the vibe changed. The home had become just a house which was ready for new life and a new family.

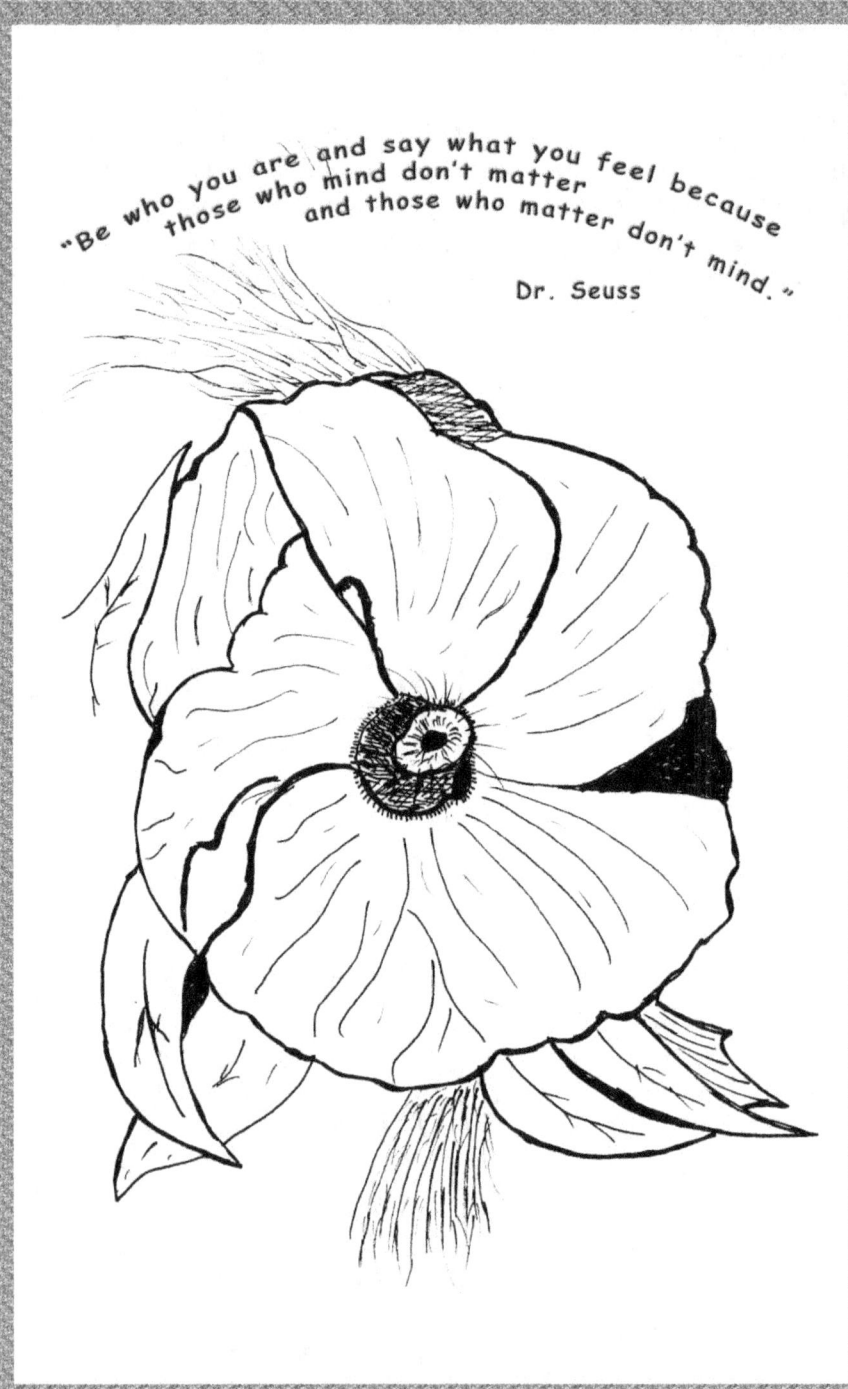

"Be who you are and say what you feel because those who mind don't matter and those who matter don't mind."

Dr. Seuss

Chapter Nine

Hindsight

As they say it is 20/20. Much clearer after you have already screwed things up! So, what would I do differently if I had it to do over again? The following are a few things I would suggest doing differently.

- Before you get to the level of full-time care, take time for yourself, vacations if you can, time off of work, whatever makes you happy and as a result stronger for the challenges ahead.
- Again, early on, allow others to assist you; later it may not be a possibility.
- If it is a possibility, consider a live-in helper with an offer of free rent or a small stipend. Family member? Maybe a person going to some level of nursing school?
- Consider the stress on others in your life, your partner or other family members. Communication and understanding are key. Good luck with that.
- Think long and hard about having a catheter placed.
- I wish I had pried more information and stories from my mother years before her memories faded and certainly before the last days when she couldn't communicate at all.
- I wish I had told my mother what an exceptional person she was, that her being in the world made a difference, not just to me but many others as well. She knew I loved her, and I would always tell her that but my fear of talking to people, particularly my mother regarding emotional thoughts, kept me from really letting her know how I felt. Too late now!
- Don't look to medical professionals to give you any real answers. There are just too many variables. Ask but do your own research and be patient. It will all happen as it is meant to be.
- Don't project. I have no idea how many wasted hours I spent worrying about what may or may not happen. Even for my

own health, I used to think, well, both grandmother and mother had hip replacements so I guess I should plan on that. Wait a minute, why should that be the case? I know I am more active, exercise more and work hard towards not having hip replacements. If you have any skeletal issues, **"Pain Free"** by *Pete Egoscue* is a great book. Simple, easy, low impact exercises that work. (Assuming you do them). My mother had AMD, oh my god what if I get that? Firstly, perhaps I am hit by a bus and never age enough to develop AMD. Secondly, what if I don't get it? How many hours did I lie awake wondering what would happen if my mother got worse and I could no longer take care of her at home? A LOT. I even spent a tremendous amount of time worrying that I wasn't doing things right or doing enough. All those wasted hours, particularly when I really needed to be sleeping. Also, let's not forget the big one that tormented me for years. What if I run out of money and can't pay the bills? Here's what I know. It all has a way of working out. Projecting about things that are in the future and are not likely to happen is a colossal waste of energy. No matter what your active mind can imagine, it isn't likely to happen that way. A book I read a long time ago suggested this solution; whatever your issue, consider the worst-case scenario, decide what you would do in that worse case scenario, then forget about it. If the worst happens, you are ready, and if, "not so worse" happens, then you can be excited about that. Despite knowing and trying this advice I still stressed about nearly everything. I really wished I could have figured worry out from the get-go and maybe I could have given my patients the best me possible rather than the stressed out, edge-on-a precipice version.

- ❖ **Patience:** You need to have a lot of this, and I don't think I had enough of it. Live in the moment. That is so easy to say and so difficult to do. I really wish I had just taken more time to just "be" with them rather than always thinking about taking care of them. That kept me from living in the moment.

- **Journal:** I kept notes here and there. If I hadn't I wouldn't have been able to write this as I wouldn't have remembered enough specifics to be useful. I have never kept a daily journal but recently, I've started writing things down. Not daily but randomly writing frustrations down somehow seems to free my mind from dwelling on them. It also prevents me from opening my mouth and causing an unnecessary argument. If I had a do-over, I think I would keep a detailed journal of my time as a caregiver. I would write about specific events as they occurred, emotions about people or events, frustrations or problems I needed to work out. I would also include at least one positive thought from the day. A gratitude moment as they say. If I hadn't ended up writing a book, perhaps I would have just used it to start a campfire and symbolically burn all the memories. Or perhaps I would have a great read about a very difficult but very special time in my life.

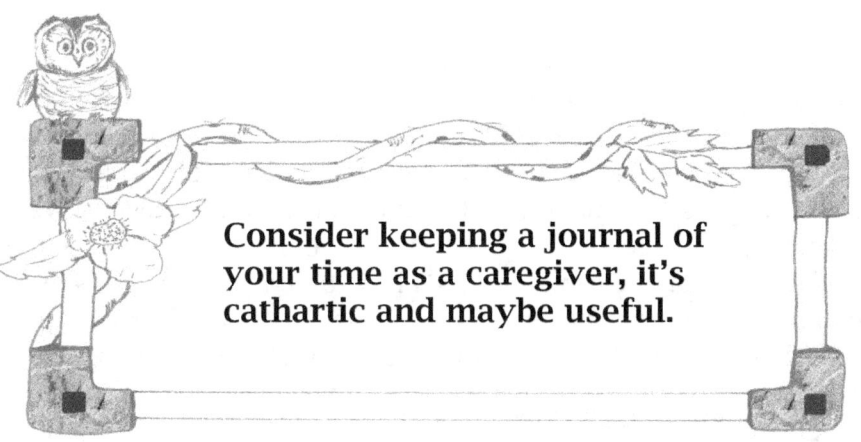

Consider keeping a journal of your time as a caregiver, it's cathartic and maybe useful.

Dog Gone It

All the same issues that we have for our people are present for our little furry friends as well. One big difference is that animals are considered property and therefore are not looked upon with the same value as people. Not trying to create a sad country song, but I also had two dogs die prior to when they should have.

The first learning experience was a dog we took in from a friend. He was a senior aged dog around eleven years old. He had a history of bad teeth and had previous tooth extractions, so I didn't think much of it. We took him to a vet that was conveniently located but was new for us. They did the extraction, we picked him up later that afternoon, but by the next day he had a lot of swelling underneath in the throat area. Long story short, turns out he had Thrombocytopenia (inability to clot) and after a blood transfusion and other efforts to save him, he died a few months after his tooth surgery. If they had tested him prior to the surgery, they would have known he had that and we would not have done the surgery.

Next dog. He was adopted from a shelter when he was around three years old. After about five years, he started to develop some bad teeth. I tried to brush them, gave him the Greenies, added the stuff to his water that was supposed to reduce the plaque, but nothing helped. Given our previous experience we were not about to have his teeth removed. However, one day he came in with a little blood spot under his eye. We thought maybe he caught it on a rose bush. We treated it with everything imaginable, but it would not heal. He also had hurt his front leg and was favoring it quite a bit, sometimes only using three legs. He was diagnosed with arthritis, and we were given a prescription for Meloxicam. The face issue was diagnosed as a tooth that was so infected it had broken through the skin and the only way to heal it would be to remove it. Again, not wanting to go there, we tried antibiotics first. Still no change. We made the difficult decision to have him undergo a dental surgery. He was tested and his blood work was in good order. The overused mantra from 2020, *"due to COVID,"* the doctor was not allowing the dog owner to come in with the dog. I did speak with the tech who answered the phone and tried to convey my concerns noting my previous experience. She indicated that the doctor would be apprised. In the forms I filled out, I also indicated that I wanted the Vet to be very conservative in treatment. Despite that, she removed 11 teeth. Not sure about you, but I don't think that is conservative. The first couple of days he was groggy but doing ok. Then he stopped eating and drinking and had difficulty getting up from a sitting position. I don't know if the Meloxicam or antibiotics had anything to do with his going downhill, but I stopped giving him anything. Called the vet but they were not helpful. I could bring him back in to have him reevaluated, but it was unlikely anything to do with his surgery, so they said. He started to have seizures; he couldn't walk on his own. He was only nine pounds to begin with now he was about six or seven. He lost control of his bladder and wouldn't drink water. We made the heart wrenching decision to let him go. In the few hours we waited for our appointment, he screeched in pain several times. If you have a pet, you can just imagine the feeling. Icing on the cake was that again, due to COVID, only one of us could go in with him. I won't even bother to say what I feel about that. The point of this story is just to reiterate that we need to ask more questions, not assume that any surgery is a simple procedure. Research the drugs prescribed and realize that all life is precious, and we shouldn't waste any time. We have to enjoy our loved ones because we just don't know what time we have. The other point is that we HOPED having his tooth removed would extend his life. We hoped and ended up making a decision we regretted.

Backup Quarterback

You know how the backup quarterback trains and yet almost never gets to play? The following year after my mother passed, my partner became a caregiver of elderly parents. Two of them. The father needed more care than what the mother could handle. I had trained for this! I had answers and could be sooo helpful. Didn't happen quite like I thought. Not only wasn't I in the game but a few times I was told my "counsel" was not needed. I was only in the beginning stages of writing this and almost threw in the towel at that point. I thought, do I really have anything of value to say or how could I help anyone if my partner wasn't even "helped." What I decided is that everyone has something of value to share and if by me sharing what I learned can help even one person or family, then it was worth the time and energy spent.

So even though I thought I would be more hands on or lead (because of my vast knowledge), I really was the backup, just there mostly for moral support or in case of emergency. And it was great to not be in charge, a break from the caregiver role. If I think about the cleat on the other foot, I wouldn't have wanted anyone to take charge or tell me how to take care of my patients. It is great to be the backup. (Not as many cuts and scrapes!)

Special Purpose

Not long after my mother passed, my friend and a fellow caregiver asked me, "So, now that you don't have, well, you know, a purpose, what are you going to do?" After a few moments with knitted brow, I said, "I am not sure, but I think I will figure something out." It would be easy to think that caring for others was my purpose in this life and I absolutely did it to the best of my abilities and was honored to do so. But that wasn't/isn't my purpose, it was just what I did. A great quote by Pablo Picasso: *"The meaning of life is to find your gift. The purpose of life is to give it away"*. So that is what I do now, whether it is art, knowledge, or time, I try to give/share as much as possible.

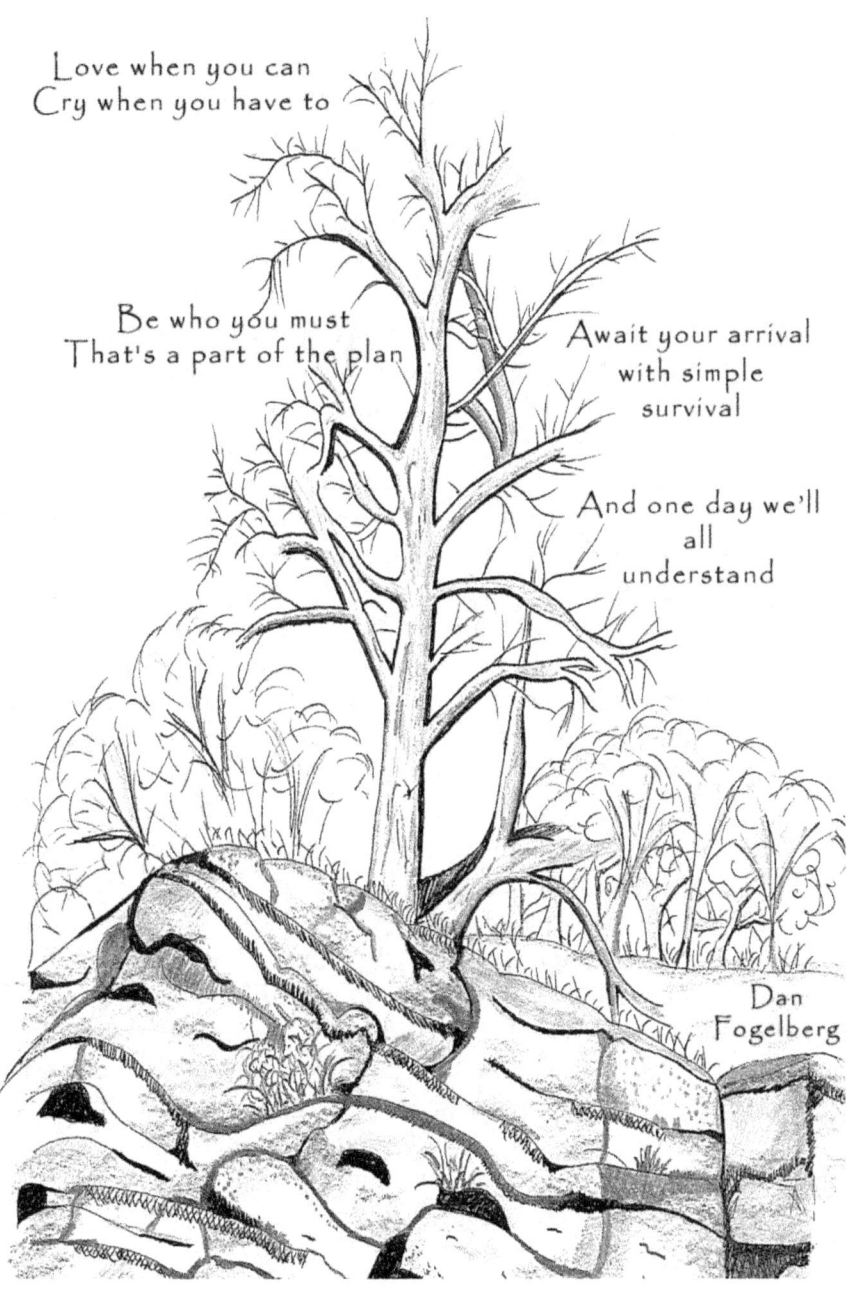

Chapter Ten

Final Thoughts

Hope is a powerful force. People can endure unbelievable atrocities and scale insurmountable hurdles because they have hope of something in the future. But hope can be deceptive as it can propel us to do things that are not necessarily the best choice. Or to take desperate measures that make things worse. Without hope it seems there is nothing to strive for, no motivation, nothing to look forward to. Unfortunately, no matter how much hope we have, nothing in life is promised. We are not guaranteed any specific number of days to live or how. Once while I was giving blood at the Red Cross, I was talking to the phlebotomist regarding the exercising that I did. I believe he was from Croatia so in his accent, he said, "You know, everyone has a finite number of heart beats so don't be in a hurry to use them up." I don't have any idea if that is true, but it is certainly an interesting thought. What if nothing we do makes any difference? If we can all avoid thinking we have any control over the future, it would sure save a lot of grief.

Since you have chosen to read this book, I assume that you find yourself in the caregiving role and likely you are or will experience that hope declines and eventually ceases to exist. Life in many ways is like a novel and as the author of your novel, you find that the story has changed, the characters changed, the vibe of the story is different, you are now different, but ultimately you are still the author. I believe it is important to create the life that ***you*** love. Not that you don't care for others, but you are the only one that knows who you are and how you want your story to go. Make that happen and others will recognize the strength, power, and positive energy that you possess and ultimately fit into your story almost as if you had written them in that way. And should you find yourself caregiving yet again, you will be better at it because you will have cared for yourself first.

I really appreciate the time you have taken to read this. My hope is that you have found something helpful for you or perhaps something you can share with others. As this book is printed on demand, I can update or alter it as needed. If you have a suggestion or comment you would like to share, please feel free to drop me an email. Please keep in mind that all I have conveyed is my story and may not ring true for you. As with everything we read, hear, or watch, take what works for you and leave the rest, investigate your own truths and as OBI Won said,

"May the force be with you."

Email: hopedeclines@yahoo.com

Additional copies of this book are available on Amazon.com

Suggested Reading

An American Sickness, How Healthcare Became Big Business and How You Can Take It Back; Elizabeth Rosenthal

Knocking On Heaven's Door
 Kay Butler

Quackery, A Brief History of the Worst Ways To Cure Everything
 Lydia Kang, MD

A Crack In Creation
 Jennifer Doudna

The Unwinding of the Miracle
 Julie Yip Williams

Stuff, Compulsive Hoarding, and the Meaning of Things
 Randy Fost and Gail Stekette

The Four Agreements and all subsequent books
 Don Miguel Ruiz, Don Jose Ruiz, Don Miguel Ruiz Jr.

On Death and Dying
 Elizabeth Kubler-Ross

Pain Free
A Revolutionary Method For Stopping Chronic Pain
 Pete Egoscue

The Power of Now or other titles
 Eckhart Tolle

The Seat of the Soul or other titles
 Gary Zukav

Links Referenced

Potential assistance with a custom ramp:
www.habitat.org/volunteer/near-you/find-your-local-habitat

Potential government assistance with eye sight loss/disability:
www.ssa.gov/benefits/ssi

Information on advanced care directives:
www.intermountainhealthcare.org/health-information/advance-directive

Reverse Mortgage information:
www.hud.gov/program_offices/housing/sfh/hcc/reverse_mortgages1

Prescription assistance through Medicare:
www.ssa.gov/benefits/medicare/prescriptionhelp.html

Prescription or health care assistance through Medicade:
www.medicaid.gov/medicaid/prescription-drugs/index.html

www.ingramcontent.com/pod-product-compliance
Lightning Source LLC
Chambersburg PA
CBHW071415210526
45465CB00001B/406